Inside this book:

- 68 joint healthy foods categorized by food group
- Eight simple tests you must try before beginning any exercise regimen
- Nine at home joint saving exercises complete with instructions and diagrams
- The popular myth and startling truth about fibromyalgia
- The real cure for misdiagnosed carpal syndrome
- A US Army-endorsed "secret" scoliosis prevention exam that takes just moments... yet no one gives
- Real-life patient tales of unnecessary surgery, overmedication, seemingly miraculous cures and other case studies

Learn what you need to know to help resolve your chronic pain problems and have a real discussion with your doctors.

CHEATING MOTHER NATURE

What You Need To Know To Beat Chronic Pain

A new tell-all book by William D. Charschan D.C., C.C.S.P.

Medical Director, USA Track and Field New Jersey
Blog Author, Diary of a NJ Chiropractor at www.backfixer1.com
www.NJLHealthandBeauty.com Health Provider
Blog Author, www.NJRunningDoc.com

This book is written to provide accurate and authoritative information with regard to the subject matter covered. It is for informational and educational purposes only. If medical advice or other assistance is required, the services of a competent professional should be sought.

Dr. William Charschan and Charschan Chiropractic and Sports Injury Associates individually or corporately, do not accept any responsibility for any liabilities resulting from the actions of any parties involved.

Dr. William D. Charschan, C.C.S.P, Charschan Chiropractic & Sports Injury Associates

ISBN: 1461128471
ISBN-13: 9781461128472

THE CAUSES OF CHRONIC PAIN ARE **<u>NOT</u>** A MYSTERY- It is Body style, Gait And Asymmetry. So why is the cure being kept a secret from you? Because doctors can't be bothered. They'd rather "medicate and move on." And frankly, most patients don't help themselves.

The truth is that chronic pain can be diagnosed visually when you know what to look for.

It's your body. For better or for worse, you are stuck with it. In sickness and in health. Isn't it time you knew the truth?

Inside this book you will learn what you need to know to resolve your pain problem and have a real discussion with your doctors including:

- 68 joint healthy foods
- 9 at home joint saving exercises
- The popular myth and startling truth about fibromyalgia
- A US Army endorsed secret scoliosis prevention examination that takes just moments… yet no one gives
- Real-life patient tales of unnecessary surgery, overmedication, seemingly miraculous cures and other case studies

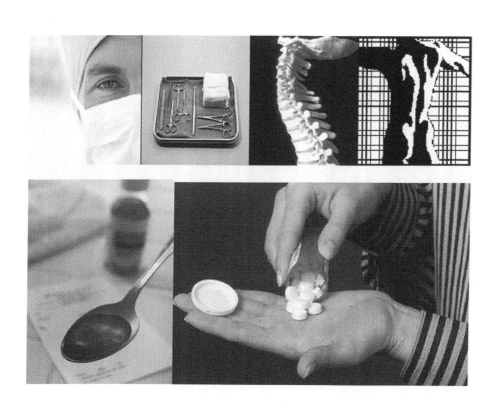

Thanks to...

Wow. The process of writing a book is incredibly different from writing and publishing an article. Not having any previous experience with this process, I needed help in organizing the subjects, making the book more compelling as I made my case and shaping the subject matter in a way that would engage and motivate the average reader to understand the issues and challenges in way that helps them better help themselves. I was fortunate to have certain well-known mentors available to me as I continued on the journey of completing this manuscript.

A special thanks to Phil Hossler, ATC. Phil has previously published texts and was able to provide guidance, helping me edit and structure my manuscript. His expertise and the time he took to help me create this book were invaluable. Thanks also to Mark Daniels of My Sales Hero LLC (http://mysaleshero.net). Mark reorganized and edited my manuscript to give it the feel and user friendliness that it needed to engage my readers and communicate my thoughts more effectively.

Thank you to Michael Leahy DC, CCSP for teaching me Active Release Techniques® his well-known method of myofascial release treatment. Additional thanks to Graston Technique, their method of instrument assisted soft tissue treatment and to Warren Hammer DC, DACBO who, in this author's opinion, wrote one of the greatest books ever on soft tissue methods keeping an objective eye to different soft tissue evaluation and treatment methods, and sharing this lovingly with his profession.

Additionally, I want to thank Professor Brian Rothbart, DPM, whose early publications on the human frame motivated me to look outside of the box of chronic pain, inspiring me to look at the problem of pain from the ground up.

A special thank you to Thomas Myers, whose book on Anatomy Trains, willingly and bravely challenges the status quo of our limited understanding of the fascial system and introduces new information with the potential to make the treatment of musculoskeletal care much more effective.

There are others that over the years influenced my strive for greatness in my profession of chiropractic such as Tom Hyde DC, DACBO, Phil Santiago DC, DACBO and too many more to name here as well as each of my patients. To all of the unnamed, please accept my apologies and my sincere gratitude for your influence and help in shaping my practice and this book.

Of course, my loving wife Beth deserves the greatest thanks for putting up with my constant obsession with the book, with the title, with getting it right and above all, by just being Beth.

Healthcare in the United States is excessively expensive and needs a change that is more creative, yields better outcomes with less risk and lower costs while satisfying the needs of the our public (our patients, of course), without who we as providers would not exist. Providers of health care should be motivated to get the best and fastest result and the systems within which we work should get out of the way, allowing good health care providers to do their jobs, without the interference of profit motivated third party payers.

Ultimately, the public wins or loses depending on our motivations and our expertise as providers. Currently there are too many snake oil salespersons in healthcare using fear to motivate people to have expensive procedures performed or to take dangerous medications with little benefit or negative consequences resulting from their methods. In my opinion, our public should always be the winners with effective and competent healthcare.

Foreword

At some point 'enough is enough'.

When was the last time you *sincerely* asked a friend, sibling or parent, "How are you?" and wanted an honest answer? If you are like most people, you are afraid that innocent greeting launches you into a twenty-three minute discussion about aches, pains, doctor's diagnoses, medications, scheduled surgery and endless health care insurance nightmares that only add to the stress and anxiety of the loved one; when all you wanted to hear was, "Great. Thanks. How about you?" It's okay to admit it.

The problem is that you and I really do have pain problems and want someone to listen.

Every night, millions of us sit around the dinner table, generationally sandwiched between our children and our parents, listening to medical and financial woes. We have lunch with our contemporaries just waiting for the right time and searching for the right way to bring up medically related issue in the hopes someone has lived through something similar and lived to tell the tale, wizened with advice and recommendations.

Millions of people suffer from chronic pain in their neck, back and joints.

- Chronic back, neck, shoulder, arm, hand, knee and foot/ankle pain may be avoided by simple screening procedures the army routinely does (army regulation 40-501).

- This same procedure should be used when you are screened for scoliosis in school.

- Addressing causes early enough can help prevent chronic pain, joint breakdown in the ankles, knees, hips, shoulders and spine.

- There are health care providers who look at function rather than just your symptoms, who can be much more helpful in resolving many painful conditions.

Because of an unacceptable level of discomfort, some knowingly, and most unknowingly, suffer from inadequate sleep. These weary travelers through life's day suffer from more than the obvious pains they tolerate. Work suffers. Intimacy is less than a passing thought. Family fun time with the kids is a tedious checkmark on the list of 'things I have to do'.

> • Too many people needlessly suffer from painful joints and interrupted sleep often wrongly classified as Fibromyalgia when their problem is mechanical and not systemic.

Amateur and professional athletes repeatedly strain muscles, even when they believe they have followed the best advice and properly stretched and warmed up.

The vast majority of people suffering from chronic shoulder and back pain problems aren't even aware they are surrounded by family who suffer from the same issues... especially as they age.

You and I inherit more than our family's good looks. You and I inherit the way we are built. We inherit the way we stand. We inherit the way we walk. We pick up the habits of our chronically suffering relatives, unconsciously changing how we do things to cope with problems of which we are not yet aware, adapting to our surroundings largely due to the mechanics of our individually inherited body styles. Recently on March 7, 2011, the NY Times reported that back pain really does run in families (http://www.nytimes.com/2011/03/08/health/08really.html?_r=1) and increasing evidence shows back pain is a family trait.

Chronic Pain is a Functional Problem Requiring Functional Solutions

Chronic pain is a matter of poor function requiring fundamental functional solutions. Widespread patient frustration with chronic pain has and continues to lead to expensive tests, surgeries, medications and other treatments that typically address a single symptom rather than provide significant and lasting relief of all the symptoms.

This book is for anyone who ever:
- Got an unsatisfactory answer from his physician.
- Received a prescription instead of a solution.
- Went through a course of injections or treatments that only worked for a short time.
- Received a massive and largely incomprehensible bill from a health insurance company.

This book is for anyone who is sick and tired of promised cures that are expensive and simply don't work.

In this book, you explore why some people have problems and why others do not. You will learn how a functional approach, rather than a symptoms based approach provides the best chances of finding the most effective health care provider and fixing a problem rather than masking a symptom.

If you have ever suffered from pain in the neck, shoulders, mid and lower back, feet, knees and hips, use this book to empower yourself to find the most effective solutions to your problems. This book is written to help you understand your body in a way you won't find on the bookshelves today. Understanding why you are in pain and how a functional evaluation and solution is more likely to help than the traditional symptoms based medical training most doctors receive will better arm you in your fight against pain and give you a fighting chance to experience a better quality of life.

The Enlightened Practitioner

In this book, you will read about the "Enlightened Practitioner". This refers to the rare individuals in the health care professions who listen and look beyond the patient complaints, the obvious symptoms, and his or her symptom-disease based training to search out and implement real answers to the real problems you experience every day.

The enlightened practitioner is the physician whose scientific approach includes looking at <u>function</u> rather than just the symptoms, thereby virtually assuring a greater likelihood that the prescribed method of treatment will resolve your problem.

Maybe reading this book will help you or a loved one find him, her, or them...

Dr. William Charschan

Table of Contents

SECTION I

Your Health Care System

Designed to Limit Choices

No one can argue that the U.S. health care system needs a thorough reevaluation. Government policy makers have been looking at the problem since President Franklin Pierce in 1854. In 1912, President Theodore Roosevelt supported universal coverage. Presidents Franklin D. Roosevelt, Truman, Johnson, Nixon, Ford, Carter, Reagan, Clinton, both Bushes and Obama made health care reform a 'priority' for their administrations[1].Of course, we all know that during each administration something always 'comes up'. Lawmakers get distracted by other pressing issues or are unable to agree upon or make the 'sweeping change', and instead settle for small changes while publicizing big victories.

Unfortunately, this lack of progress continues to hit home hard, especially this far into the new millennia. We can no longer afford the most outrageously expensive health care system in the world where care is economically rationed, causing the average American to put off care because he cannot afford it due to high out of pocket costs even with insurance. (http://www.nytimes.com/2010/08/17/health/policy/17health. html?_r=1.).

● Too many people with serious illnesses suffer financial hardships in the U.S. at the hands of an overpriced system that offers little benefit per dollar compared to systems that exist in other countries.

We simply cannot tolerate a system that bankrupts families and delivers care that is more expensive, and in many ways is inferior, than that which other countries deliver. In other countries, rather than economic rationing, the government manages health care through global budgets. The concern is that in either case, health care is rationed.

As a whole, the U.S. Managed Care System fails to deliver on the promise of effective and affordable high quality[2] care to the public. The system recklessly siphons off money for care management while unsympathetically limiting care within a dysfunctional and disconnected health care management paradigm. It has failed over the years to weed out unnecessary procedures, interventional measures (which have no benefit and are potentially   harmful) in both young and old, which have not improved the human condition. The general public has been indoctrinated into believing all this is necessary to sustain life, when in fact, it leads to higher costs which have little proven benefit for the public at large. We have seen evidence of this when we held open forums to discuss changes to our healthcare system which could eventually insure every American. We have a medical industrial complex which is simply out of control.

♦ Managed care simply rations our inefficient and bloated system by creating barriers for patients who can only access certain health care providers- unless willing to risk what can be extreme financial consequences.

But what other way is there?

♦ Well, the U.S. can take a step off the world leader pedestal long enough to look around the globe for other successful health care models that can, with a little effort, be adapted to work in the U.S. In other countries, the government rations health care insurance coverage using a global budget that selectively decides who receives which procedures, and how long he may wait.

In the current U.S. health care system, your insurance company can outright deny your doctor's request for medically necessary care forcing you to go out of your network at great personal cost to seek the provider you believe you need to solve your problem. If you cannot afford the visit, you do not go; and at some point you risk becoming an emotional drain on your family as well as a financial burden to both your family and society.

Co-payments, the share the insured person must pay to access the health care system continue to increase year to year. At the same time as your co-payment increases you, the consumer, pay more each year for health care coverage – the amount you pay for the privilege of carrying health insurance either individually or through your employer (who, incidentally continues to see his costs rise to the point of seriously considering the cost-benefit and shareholder value of remaining in business).

2010 health care legislation has made it almost illegal to either not carry or for a larger employer not to offer insurance to their workers. The decision, contested in several courts and under fire from a newly elected congress could be repealed, modified, or expanded. It is anyone's guess what condition healthcare is in by the time you are reading this book.

The one constant is that the health insurers' inability to prevent health care costs from escalating beyond the means of the average American results in an economic rationing where more of your hard-earned dollars feed a system that each year costs you more and gives you less.

To cope, people do what they can afford to do, even if it is not in their best interest[3].

But that's not even the real problem.

The Problem with Insurance and the High Cost of Care

The U.S. system of health care is prohibitively expensive compared to other systems around the world, consuming a considerable amount of our gross national product. Yet, according to the World Health Organization (WHO) it is considered inferior to the health systems in many other countries.

"Americans spend twice as much as residents of other developed countries on healthcare, but get lower quality, less efficiency and have the least equitable system," reads a June 23, 2010 article (www.Reuters. com). "U.S. Scores Dead Last in Study" headlines the article by Maggie Fox, Reuter's Health and Science Editor in reviewing the findings of the non-profit organization Commonwealth Fund study. Schoen, of the Commonwealth Fund told reporters that, "We (The U.S.) rank last on safety and do poorly on several dimensions of quality. We do particularly poorly on going without care because of cost. And we also do surprisingly poorly on access to primary care and after-hours care."

To understand why, consider for just a moment those who lack health insurance and those who are underinsured with huge out of pocket co-payments. These people are vulnerable to their health condition bankrupting them and in some cases, people have lost everything due to a significant health condition according to Reuters News Service report on a U.S. Government Study[4].

Managed Care has failed to control the true drivers of cost in our system while adding unnecessary costs of its own including paperwork, denials of appropriate care and limiting the choice of providers you can use.

Earning fair and reasonable profit for services is a fair business practice. Managed Care, however, financially strangles doctors in the name of unreasonable profit margin expectations intended to fuel growth artificially by outrageous spending on advertising and lobbying our elected officials in Washington for laws that benefit only the Managed Care industry instead of health care as a whole in our country.

Rather than having a reward for quality efficiencies (care that is most effective and appropriate for the condition), Managed Care seeks alternative ways of reducing expense, like limiting medically necessary care.

By primarily seeking cost savings through limiting medically necessary care, many specialists opt out of networks because they recognize that they are under-reimbursed in the network. Out of network, that same doctor's reimbursement levels often seem quite exaggerated in comparison.

I personally know of a neurosurgeon that was incredibly busy when he was in network. However, he had little free time for himself or his family. Eventually he opted out of all plans except for Medicare.

His volume dropped dramatically. His income, however, remains similar to when he was in the networks. He is able to maintain his financial income with less patients because his medical care niche is limited to fewer doctors in his specialty.

Unfortunately, medical specialties with more doctors usually have no choice but to participate in the networks. The insurance companies know this. They are designed for and have no issue with taking advantage of the situation.

You and I now find ourselves paying for care out-of-network that any reasonable individual agrees should be covered in the network. We find our choices limited to just the doctors in the network with our choice of specialists usually limited either by the plan, or by our primary care doctor's relationships if we are in an Health Maintenance Organization (HMO).

Every year, our premiums increase well beyond the rate of inflation with www. http://hr.blr.com/ reporting that for 2009, coverage increases of at least 10% are expected for many employers[5].

• It doesn't stop there. In the heat and confusion of an emergency, some health plans may not cover the visit if you forget to call your plan's 800 number before your emergency room visit. And it gets worse.

You are more likely than not to learn that the fee for the emergency room visit (eg: a cut that required stitches) is just one of many bills you are now responsible for paying because each doctor independently bills for the emergency room service provided. These independent invoices can quickly add up to thousands of dollars for a few minutes of time required to take care of the problem. These billing practices are outrageous because they are allowed.

And there's another way HMOs gets you.

You visit your general practitioner who orders a battery of tests conducted at a lab- not the doctor's office. Much later you find out that the lab fee is not covered because it is not the lab with whom your HMO contracts.

Or, maybe you go to an in-network physician for a medical procedure thinking the cost after co-pay and deductions is covered only to later learn that the facility or the anesthesiologist is not considered in-network.

You have to be crazy not to wonder if this is any way to run health care.

Health care Network Fee Gap Solution

Another concern is the enormous gap in cost-for-services assessed by different providers when comparing their in-network and out-of-network fees; fees that are often much more generous to out of network providers. Fees that are frankly ridiculous for the work actually being performed.

Instead, consider the following 'regional fair fee' solution.

It would be much more equitable if health care plans paid one regionally based service fee whether the physician or facility is in or out of the network. The idea of a fair regionally-based reimbursement system that treats every provider as though he or she is in-network can be the ideal behind a national health care system.

Think about it. Given the option, wouldn't you want a health care system that is well integrated and effective? One that is fiscally prudent? One with less administrative paperwork and restrictions? One that rewards preventive behavior? One where everyone is covered? I know I would.

"I will apply, for the benefit of the sick, all measures [that] are required...[.]

I will remember that there is art to medicine as well as science, and that warmth, sympathy, and understanding may outweigh the surgeon's knife or the chemist's drug.

I will prevent disease whenever I can, for prevention is preferable to cure.

- *Exceprts from the Modern Hyppocratic Oath; source: www.medterms.com*

Of course, you have to get past the rabid shouts of 'socialism' from the far right and look past the political noise suggesting this idea is socialistic and instead accept that the real purpose of health care is to provide medical help to a person who requires it. The real purpose of health care is to provide medical care to a person to help overcome illness whenever possible.

Make no mistake. I accept, and so should you, that health care is a big business for doctors, drug companies and hospitals. It therefore needs a big business mindset.

Health care can learn something from a successful non-healthcare business model where the focus is on the customer.

That's right. Health care should not be about the doctors, the drug companies and the hospitals. Ultimately and always it should be about you, the consumer… the patient.

As a country the U.S. must look at why our system of care has lost its way and we must do everything we can to help it back toward its true purpose; helping and not bankrupting you when you become ill. And you as the patient and consumer can and need to be an active participant.

Prevention Versus Intervention: Obvious Health care Cost Drivers

You already know that lifestyle is one cost driver. What we eat, whether we exercise, and what we do for a living all contribute to both our health and our health issues.

Unfortunately, our current state of intervention versus prevention must be defined more clearly; in terms easily understood by everyone inside and outside the medical community; in such a way that each of us can readily accept that prevention is always less costly than intervention and then do something about it.

So, why is most of what we do in our current system interventional? With test results typically leading to interventional drugs? With treatments and tests in the *name of prevention* that lead to further procedures, drugs, and tests? Where does this all lead and does this really help solve our health related problems?

Does everyone on medication really need the medication they are on?

As a physician, I am not convinced that the root cause of blood pressure issues, cholesterol problems, osteoporosis and the many other conditions on which health care providers have you and I focus are well understood.

I am convinced, however, that big pharma has a huge stake in offering you and me lifelong subscriptions for medications to address symptoms and test results (not necessarily to resolve problems) that in the end may or may not improve your health. In fact, the medicine you are taking for one symptom can easily be the cause for a different and potentially more dangerous problem.

A casual reading of your prescriptions warning labels advises you that many of these medications can and *do* cause side effects that require monitoring to prevent serious complications. Cholesterol medications are a classic example because they can cause liver and muscle damage, as many of my patients over the years can attest.

Still, the Centers for Disease Control reported in 2006 that, "...medications were ordered or provided in over two-thirds of the 1.1 billion visits to physician offices." Prescribing drugs is obviously central to how physicians treat patients; and by extension, critical to pharmaceutical companies. But is it necessary? Is it right? Is it really health care?

You have to ask if the benefits outweigh the risks.

You also have to ask something else…

Rather than prescribing more tests, medication and surgery to pull test results back in line, shouldn't doctors search out and treat the root cause of high blood pressure, bone loss, and cholesterol problems?

My friend calls this "Alice in Wonderland Medicine", after the scenes in both the original Lewis Carroll book and classic Disney cartoon movie where Alice experiments, eating and drinking different amounts of biscuits and liquid to achieve her desired height (take this to bring your numbers up; take this to lower your numbers). You may recall that each nibble and each sip caused Alice a problem worse than the existing problem she was trying to solve until she finally got it just right.

As a whole, the U.S. spends more per capita than any other country in the world for health care. Still, our population can hardly be called healthy when compared to many other industrialized nations. Particularly as the cost of offering benefits continues to rise forcing employers to cut health care benefits[6]. Many smaller employers have entirely stopped carrying health insurance benefit plans.

Disease Method of Treatment

also

Symptons Evaluation:

Diagnosing and treating a pathological symptom that is not the direct result of a physical injury.

Health care reform is trying to change this, forcing small employers and individuals to carry insurance or face stiff taxes and fines. This is not a solution. Making someone pay for something that he stopped paying for because he cannot afford it sounds more like an Abbott and Costello routine than health care reform.

Death May be Easier Than Comedy. It isn't Cheaper.

New Jersey, my home state, was recently named the most expensive place to die in the country[7]. This is because the system values longevity with intervention vs. quality of life. Defying all logic, the continuation of expensive procedures while one is dying instead of just offering hospice or home care and palliative comfort care during the patient's last days is more common than the average person realizes.[8]

In 2009 it was reported that in New Jersey a hospice care facility often gets a dying patient 17 days before death versus 30 days in other states because the patient required their last session of chemotherapy[9].

Seriously?! Did the patient really need his last session of chemo if he is unresponsive to the care and is dying? So much for death with dignity.

Blame the Symptom Model Ideology

Our health care system is broken. It is broken because of the symptom-model ideology and the seeming lack of ethics regarding decisions about who should and who should not live based entirely on expensive technology capable of prolonging existence. All without considering your quality of life concerns after the intervention is performed.

Recently, a patient revealed to me that her 89 year-old mom, a very sharp person, had a heart valve problem. Her mom was going to die unless she had open-heart surgery. I expressed concern that at her mom's age, and overall physical condition, that she was likely not going to survive the surgery; and even if she did, her quality of life would ultimately be in doubt.

This obviously was a hard decision. Emotion overrides common sense. The natural instinct and will to live often drives people to opt for the surgery, only to die a horrible death anyway. In this woman's case, her surgery resulted in countless problems: rehab, body systems shutting down, poorly healing wounds, infections. Sadly, she is living out her days in a nursing home, unable to take care of herself any longer, with a poor quality of life.

The option taken resulted in a horrible experience, exhausting the patient's finances, depleting her Medicare benefits, and taking its toll on her family, only to watch their loved one die an undignified death.

Was it really appropriate to have supplied this choice when this was clearly not a good or even fair option for the patient. Was this option medically ethical?

The better option would have been counseling, making her as comfortable as possible and preparing her and her family for the inevitable. This story is just one example of what is wrong. Had there been no Medicare to pay the bill, the patient likely never would have been given the surgery option in the first place.

One has to ask, was this ever a viable health care procedure to benefit the patient, or a financial decision for the benefit of the doctors and the facility?

We spend years and countless dollars training specialists to evaluate our bodies with a 'disease mentality'; and to diagnose a person as if he is not the sum of his or her parts. This is known also as 'symptoms evaluation'.

On the surface it sounds okay. Right? Yet, symptoms evaluation leads to testing that leads to expensive procedures that are all expensive because they are designed to be expensive. You can call it the medical industrial complex if you will.

Would it surprise you to learn that only a small portion of these tests truly gives us the answers we desire? *I don't doubt this!*

Most medical specialists know little about the musculoskeletal system, yet the musculoskeletal system often imitates many organ based system problems and visa versa.

How much do you want to bet that if your medical practitioner better understood how to evaluate the musculoskeletal system and was offered a better incentive for a more thorough evaluation and the quality time spent with you instead of a high reimbursement for procedures to diagnose symptoms, that most medical specialists would order fewer tests?

Want to bet that if your primary physician better understood how to evaluate the musculoskeletal system, he would also more readily and more appropriately refer you to other classes of providers who can treat the musculoskeletal problem that is really creating the symptom?

Unnecessary testing and a woeful lack of manual diagnostic skills combined with fear of financially crippling litigation create a huge cost driver in our health care system.

Sometimes More Is Less. Sometimes Less Is More.

Admittedly, there are times when seemingly more expensive interventions cost less in the long run. And there are a significant number of instances when less is more.

Many studies show that states with a higher number of primary care general practitioners and fewer numbers of specialists experience lower overall costs of care. Fewer specialists means fewer procedures and overall lower costs[10].

One Illinois study used chiropractors in an HMO as primary care physicians[11]. The study shows a high patient-customer satisfaction ranking, markedly lower costs compared to typical medical management via fewer interventions, fewer hospitalizations as well as less a much lower utilization of drugs.

Perhaps it is time our health care system re-examines and re-evaluates the current paradigm, and decides what primary care actually is, and who is most capable of providing the service.

The Cost of a Chemically-Dependent Society

Forget marijuana and cocaine. Managing every complaint and symptom with another medication is another major health care cost driver[12].

Almost conspiratorially working together, our health care system and large pharmaceutical consumer products companies and wildly creative and successful advertising agencies created a chemically dependent society trained to take drugs in the absence of real cures and solutions to real problems.

Look at it this way. Under our current health care model, practically every problem requires a prescription medication. For each prescription medication you take, your pharmacist is expected to talk with your doctor to make sure there isn't a life-threatening interaction of different drugs and your doctor has to monitor you to make sure the medication is either not interfering nor negatively reacting with the other medications you take.

Statins, cholesterol medications, are good examples of this. In many people, statins destroy muscle tissue and creates problems in other body systems[13]. Doctors must monitor patients on these medications closely to prevent a life-threatening event.

Still, there is another concern with the long term and very real human side effects of this approach. We are living longer. Many of us, Baby Boomers, find we are in the difficult position of caring for both our children and our parents. How many of our seniors, our parents, in their late 80's and early 90's really need all the prescribed medication they take, or the tests and procedures which are ordered for them? Is there any substantial proof the medications they take improve their quality of life? Is there any substantial proof they need all those procedures or tests, as if their doctor will be able to extend their lives and their quality of life indefinitely?

We Do a Couple Things Right. But We Could Do So Much More.

On the other hand, the U.S. health care system has some of the best emergency medicine in the world. Countless lives are saved from heart attacks, debilitating strokes, and other problems.

Unfortunately, this excellent react and respond care is just a small part of our health care system, with the majority of chronic health problems using the prescription drug model because real and permanent solutions do not exist or are not being researched.

A convincing case can be made that cures are neither researched nor found because companies and shareholders understandably feel strongly about the less effective, faster-to-market and easier-to-market more profitable alternatives. Said another way, curing a problem is not nearly as financially rewarding for a drug company's revenue model as regularly treating a symptom for extended periods of time.

A case can be made for government research for many problems like cancer where a corporation's efforts may be less than whole-hearted as a cure could put a big dent in a corporation's long-term revenue stream.

What the system can't take to the bank is largely ignored.

A real-life example of this is the diagnosis of H Pylori for stomach ulcers[14]. An Italian doctor theorized and executed his theory on duodenal ulcers over a period of more than twenty years. He was ignored for many more years because it was more profitable to have people subscribe to Tagamet® and other drugs instead of allowing a cure that would cut off the revenue flow from the drugs sold.

A patient typically takes Tagamet® 4 times a day, from 4 to 12 weeks in the short-term and can be on a maintenance level prescription for up to five years. A patient taking the drug exposes himself to a variety of side-effects that may include headache, mental confusion, agitation, psychosis, depression, anxiety, hallucinations, disorientation, development of breasts in males, impotence, in rare cases anaphylaxis, hypersensitivity vasculitis (inflammation of the blood vessels), bradycardia (slow heart rate), tachycardia (fast heart rate) and heart block. Other rare and debilitating musculoskeletal side effects can include arthralgia (joint pain), myalgia (muscle pain), polymositis (generalized muscle inflammation) and a worsening of joint symptoms in arthritis patients[15].

> Tagamet®- Almost all of the side effects are categorized as reversible. But, should you really have to expose yourself to additional problems?

How about a 10¢ cancer cure?

I know it sounds outrageous, and 10 cents is a bit of an exaggeration, however the Italian doctor mentioned earlier, T. Simoncini, thinks he has found the cause and cure for most cancers. He believes that Candida Albicans, a fungus almost always found present in cancer patients is the cause of the cancer mutating cells, rather than a result of the mutated cancerous genes[16].

For twenty years he has treated these tumors with bicarbonate (baking soda). As you might imagine, he is fighting an uphill battle against more popular acceptance by not just the U.S. health care system since you cannot justify an inflated price for baking soda, and a ridiculous cost for administering the cure.

According to this source, the statistical survival rates for chemo patients and radiation therapy are not anywhere nearly as favorable as most people believe despite the reputations of institutions such as Sloan Kettering whose business model would implode if a true solution was actually found.

The fight to stay alive with these methods is horrible. Patient white cells are eradicated in the hopes of killing the cancer with side-effects that include hair loss, weakness, nausea and more from poisoning the body. I know few oncologists who administer this to patients who would like to experience this treatment themselves.

Therefore, it is surprising that while managed care companies claim to be so interested in realizing huge cost savings and improving the quality of care for cancer patients that they have not looked more seriously into methods like this bicarbonate treatment. It has the earmark of a cost effective method for treatment that the government should be much more interested in researching and testing.

This is just another reason government-run health care in the United States may not be such a bad idea.

There is hope, though. You can visit www.curenaturalicancro.com and download the 2009 research article written by several doctors from

U.S. cancer research organizations based in Arizona and Florida who tested the bicarbonate solution. The 9-page report is titled: "Bicarbonate Increases Tumor pH and Inhibits Spontaneous Metastases" and can be found here:

http://www.curenaturalicancro.com/pdf/bicarbonate-increases-tumor-ph-and-inhibits-metastases.pdf.

The Cost of Trafficking Body Parts

In our current health care paradigm, doctors evaluate pain and assume it is the problem. Sadly, the typical health care practitioner does not fully evaluate or consider the importance of body mechanics as the ultimate cause for painful conditions.

Not surprisingly, the typical health care practitioner concerns himself mainly with the disease and the injury. He approaches the symptomatic problem from his own point of view.

Take for example scoliosis screening. It's ironic how we routinely screen for scoliosis in schools but ignore potential issues caused by body mechanics that can be improved with a simple insert in your child's shoes. These are issues that later in life result in chronic foot, ankle, knee, hip, lower back, upper back, shoulder and neck pain.

Checking your children's feet during scoliosis screening would take just one more minute and offer a developing adolescent the promise of a better quality of life. Before you go thinking this requires a lot of background and training you should know that it is an easy test. Athletic trainers, nurses as well as other health professionals within the school system are already qualified and willing to perform these screens, yet, don't.

Instead, we spend billions of dollars annually replacing bad knees, hips and treating the symptoms of poor body mechanics that presents itself as chronic pain in joints throughout our bodies.

Unfortunately, in our health care system, there are many who would like to keep the status quo because this is where the money is.

Companies who make prosthetics that replace our original body parts advertise with the drug companies during prime time television to get the public to use their products in the replacement. The non-medical public, as well as your primary care physicians, seem convinced that body parts just go bad. Like car parts...

And what do you do when a part goes bad? Replace it, of course.

If the assertion that body parts just wear out is true, why do so many people live their lives fully, without ever having a body part wear out or go bad to the point it needs replacing? What is different about the people who do wear out their joints?

This question is the elephant in the room and is why we must screen our children for genetic tendencies toward poor function. We can save many people from debilitating chronic pain, unnecessary surgery, superfluous medication and needless suffering by screening our children when they are young using the same simple criteria the army uses when assessing a recruit[17].

Kinetic Chain:

The series of connected muscles, ligaments, nerves and joints relating to producing motion.

The current health care system is out of touch with the realities of function and is missing out on an opportunity to truly help people age better.

Later in this book, in the "You" Section, you will gain a better understanding of how this works. For now, just accept the premise that you cannot isolate knee pain from hip pain or from foot pain. Your health care provider must evaluate the entire kinetic chain, not just the symptomatic area. The lower kinetic chain is a series of joints (ankle, knee and hip) that must be evaluated together.

Not understanding kinetic chains, how they work, how they produce pain when they dysfunction and the ramifications of not identifying these problems early in life has created hundreds of thousands of people who suffer needlessly- just because of the way they are built.

Until we experience a change in the current health care paradigm we cannot significantly lower the cost, the suffering and improve people's lives sufficiently and cost effectively.

An Unbiased Opinion on Back Treatment- the May 2009 Consumer Reports

A multi-billion dollar problem, lower back pain syndromes continue to tax the system. There are many, many suggested solutions. Can they all be right?

There are an endless number of specialists who all want to treat lower back pain patients and just as many different forms of treatments. These can include physical therapy, chiropractic (one of the oldest and proven effective beginning with bone setting going back thousands of years), back surgery, epidural injections, exercise regimens, medications, and more.

A Badly Broken System

Evaluate the Symptom

Apply Treatment To the Symptom

Run Tests

Visit Specialist/ Surgeon When Problem Is Not Resolved

The reality is that there is a lot of money being made in back pain treatment, and nobody wants to give up his or her piece of the pie.

The May 2009 issue of Consumer Reports, published a patient satisfaction survey regarding providers who treat back pain and back pain relief remedies[18].

Among the many providers and proposed solutions considered, the report was highly favorable across the globe for manipulation performed primarily by Chiropractors and occasionally by Osteopathic physicians with Chiropractors cited most often when spinal manipulation for back treatment is considered.

Consumer Reports cautioned against the use of narcotics, most often the prescribed cocktail of muscle relaxers and anti-inflammatory medications commonly used when primary care and specialist medical providers manage back pain.

Primary care physician satisfaction rating with treating back pain was only 34%; while specialist medical physicians were slightly better at 44%.

The highest satisfaction was with chiropractic care at 59%.

It's not too surprising, really. Fifteen years earlier, in 1994, the Agency for Health care Policy and Research (AHCPR) studied back pain literature and concluded three things are effective for lower back pain. They included simply manipulation, ice and aspirin[19].

The Cost of Self-Serving Lobbyists

As you may expect, the medical-surgical lobby did not like the finding. It was not good for business and their personal interests. So the medical-surgical lobbied to cut the AHCPR funding. The lobby won, making it impossible for the AHCPR, a government agency, to continue publishing and publicizing these types of objective studies to benefit the public[20].

This is just one of the many reasons we still do not have cohesive treatment systems for lower back pain. It gets better (or worse).

Later, The American Medical Association (AMA) released its own literature that totally eliminated anything they believed competed with their methods of back treatment- including chiropractic manipulation[21].

Recently, the AMA attempted to draft legislation to eliminate the use of the term "physician" to any health care providers other than a Medical Doctor (MD) and Osteopathic Doctor (OD) in a monopolizing and anti-competitive attempt to own the health care landscape[22].

The financial motive and the willingness to stamp out competition continues to exist everywhere in health care, keeping costs high, leaving people wondering about what works and whom to trust. That's business. But, is it ethical to deny the public better care because of these health care groups self interests?

The Cost of Flawed Treatment Studies

Many studies of different treatments of back pain are flawed because they attempt to evaluate the effects of back pain treatment without truly understanding what lower back pain is. Lower back-pain treatment studies merely attempt to evaluate a treatment on a symptom, and then evaluate the effectiveness of the method of treatment.

Often, due to design, the study limits what the practitioner may do in the public samples used for the study. For example, studies may evaluate a series of manipulations on back pain to see if this gives a better outcome than exercises or massage.

In the real world, a practitioner may use manipulation, massage or other muscle and joint related treatments and exercises during the course of care to assure the desired outcome.

The good news is that even with the flaws that exist in many studies, spinal manipulation generally shows that it is more effective than other methods[23, 24].

Manipulation, most commonly performed on patients by Chiropractors, directly addresses the faulty mechanical function in the lower back, improving joint function that is important for relief.

Don't get too excited, though. Even manipulation of both the joints and muscles and ligaments in the lower back does not truly address the complete problem of lower back pain. Manipulation does, however, restore

> **Gait:**
> The way you walk, run or move on foot.

mobility and the actual act of manipulation relieves pain. Why?

Manipulation restores normal functional integrity to joints distorted by poor body mechanics, asymmetry and compensation.

I will explain more about the relationship of the lower extremity and typical gait related pain syndromes in detail later in the book. For now, understand that when we work our way up the body from the feet to the pelvis, we can see that abnormal gait patterns will involve the pelvis and create many long-term problems for people.

Another Costly Medical Mistreatment

The American Academy of Family Physicians (AAFP) web site published what they agreed upon as the common methods of evaluation and treatment for carpal tunnel syndrome. The AAFP agrees that treatment includes wrist splints that limit motion to avoid exacerbation.

You can read the report yourself: www.aafp.org/afp/20030715/265. html.

Of course, you and I know it is not a cure. The problem still exists. The point of typical splinting methods is to experiment until the best result is achieved.

The reality is like you saying, "Hey Doc, it hurts when I do this."

And your doctor replies, "So, don't do it."

This kind of knee-jerk response behavior is just neatly boxing you into your symptoms and limiting your activity with pain avoidance using a splint.

In over twenty years of clinical experience I have seen many splinted patients get worse over time because the true problem causing pain and numbness continues to exist and is not understood or addressed.

The AAPF writes about different medications used that are no better than placebos (sugar pills), including NSAID-type medications prescribed every day!

There was one study where Prednisone was found to be effective... but what about the side effects and what occurs when you stop taking it, especially after long-term usage?

You have to wonder what is the criterion used to call a treatment or procedure effective.

Does it mean fewer symptoms while on the medication? Better mobility or improved function long term without pain?

According to the AAFP article, splinting and medications reduces symptoms only and does not address the mechanical causes of the condition. Injection does not have good studies supporting it unless used with Prednisone. Carpal tunnel release surgery is recommended when non-invasive symptom relief regimens do not work and surgery works better than splinting.

Unfortunately, the article's only focus is the area of symptoms rather than concerning itself with understanding the mechanical malfunction that created the problem. While there is a small discussion of the side effects of surgery, it is interesting to note there is very little mention of other successful methods of treatment, including myofascial release.

You are starting to see the pattern. When there is no attempt to understand why the condition occurred, and physicians look only at the symptomatic part, many people receive recommendations to have an invasive procedure directed at the area of symptoms. This may seemingly relieve the symptoms for short while, but it leaves the malfunction intact.

For years, this has been the accepted approach, causing many to suffer with other biomechanically-based pain processes because the true mechanical problem is never addressed. Let me illustrate.

> A married, female patient in her mid-thirties is diagnosed with Carpal tunnel syndrome. With no improvement after splinting, various shots and prescription medications over a period of 4 – 6 weeks, and finally a Neuro Conduction Velocity (NCV) test, her doctor convinces her she needs surgery.
>
> Meanwhile, a few years earlier, she had a right lower back problem that supposedly went away.
>
> A year before that, she had a knee problem on her left side that also 'went away.'
>
> One year after the Carpal tunnel surgery, she has shoulder pain in the left side and cannot move her neck for several days.

By understanding that these conditions are all related and by understanding the mechanisms behind the pain, these problems may not have occurred. Moreover, our married mother of two may have avoided the surgery.

Her problems did not stop there. Years later, when her children are in high school, she is told she is arthritic.

These additional problems may have been prevented had her diagnosing physician understood, or referred her to a specialist who understood, the mechanical dysfunction behind her pain.

The public deserves a choice: A better option.

There are many options outside traditional care available and just as many studies revealing that the public is slowly finding its way outside the traditional insurance system to access those options[25]. Rarely, however, do you ever hear about most of these options from your traditional medical provider. Although more papers are being published suggesting medical physicians develop relationships with chiropractors they trust[26].

Restless Leg Syndrome Ridiculousness

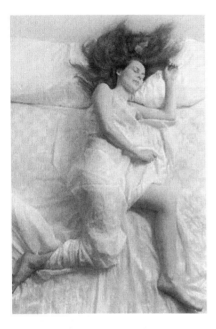

The generally accepted definition of Restless Legs Syndrome (RLS), also known as Wittmaack-Ekbom's syndrome, or sometimes referred to as Nocturnal Myoclonus, is that it is a condition characterized by an irresistible urge to move the body in an attempt to stop uncomfortable or odd sensations[27].

It gets it name because it typically affects the legs, but is known to affect the arms and torso, too. RLS causes a sensation in the legs or arms most closely compared to a burning, itching, or tickling sensation in the muscles. Moving the affected body part appears to provide temporary relief. There is some controversy surrounding the marketing of drug treatments for RLS.

Many of my patients have experienced this condition. Women, especially those who are pregnant, are prone to experience RLS (as more than just a few married men can attest), yet there does not seem to be a sound explanation as to why it occurs.

Three commonly prescribed medications are pramipexole (Mirapex), ropinirole (Requip) and rotigotine (Neupro). These drugs quiet the legs by mimicking the activity of dopamine, a molecule that acts as a hormone and a signal transmitter between cells. Such drugs are also used to treat Parkinson's disease. Side effects include nausea, dizziness, wheeziness, fatigue and transient headache.

The commonly prescribed treatment is based on the theory that RLS is neurological in nature. However, in my experience, every patient who has ever had this condition has also had problems with torsion in the pelvis.

After reading this book, you should have an understanding that gait imbalances will cause torsion in the pelvis or tortipelvis. This happens when the body tightens due to poor firing patterns in the front on one side and the back on the other. The legs, then, naturally will tighten over time as your core (mid section of your body) becomes compromised from the tightening of the surrounding myofascia.

This sounds silly, but the person will feel discomfort in the upper body as well as in the lower body when at rest because as the muscles warm down, the person notices they are not lying comfortably.

In other words, their body distorts at rest. The torsion in the pelvis also causes the sacroiliac joints to create a dull ache down and throughout the legs making it difficult to get comfortable. Meanwhile, the upper body is placed under tension as the pelvis tightens.

I have just described symptoms, not of RLS, but of tortipelvis, or pelvis torsion. As you have just read, the symptoms of tortipelvis or pelvic torsion are very similar to restless leg syndrome. Unfortunately, most doctors will jump all over the easy but incorrect RLS diagnosis.

My patients report a significant level of relief and even resolution of the condition without medication after undergoing Myofascial Release treatment to restore normal function to the myofascia surrounding their core muscles, which include the erector spinae, multifidii, rectus abdominus and oblique muscles as well as the leg muscles.

This eliminates the need to rely on prescription medications and their inevitable side effects.

I will say it again. If the problem is mechanical in nature, how can a medication fix the problem? In reality, it appears the medical community is in a conspiracy to place someone on a medication long-term. The goal is to relieve the symptoms of the condition as long as you continue taking the medication, rather than resolve the condition.

Of course, treating any condition this way is controversial. After all, which makes more sense? Treating the symptom, or understanding the mechanics that created the problem and then treating the mechanical aberration until a more stable mechanical state that resolves the symptoms is achieved?

Re-Defining Preventive Care

This is going to sound silly. When is 'preventive' really 'preventive' vs. when does a 'preventive' screening procedure lead to an aggressive intervention that may or may not be helpful to the individual is a serious question.

Carotid Endarterectomy is a procedure that was thought to prevent strokes because it cleaned the carotid artery of clots. Unfortunately, studies show that in areas where there were more medical specialists, more procedures are recommended and performed leading to more strokes. It is a perfect example of interventional procedures designed to prevent health issues that may actually create more problems than if it is left alone in certain cases since it has been shown to have a complication rate of 6%[28].

Brushing your teeth daily is a preventive intervention that continues to show a decrease in cavities and improvement in the condition of the gums, as well as a benefit to cardiac health too[29]. Tooth care is an example of self-administered prevention that with a high degree of certainty can eliminate intervention. Just like your diet. Of course, dentists recommend periodic visits intended to improve upon the practice of brushing ones teeth, to remove deep-seated food in the gums and between teeth, the typical daily ritual misses.

Years ago, before regular dental regimens were commonplace, many people lost their teeth when they were much younger; and many more had to endure dentures. In today's society, preventive dental care helps many people keep their original teeth and regularly scheduled preventive maintenance visits uncover potential problems, which are addressed before any real damage has occurred.

Preventive care is supposed to be about making sure you stay healthy. It is not supposed to be about whether or not there should be invasive testing. That is disease process screening. Do not confuse the two.

The Cost and Concept of Prevention and Preventive Care

Has anyone ever defined preventive care satisfactorily?

Wikipedia defines preventive care as "a set of measures taken in advance of symptoms to prevent illness or injury. This type of care is best known by routine physical examinations and immunizations. The emphasis is on preventing illnesses before they occur."

In our health care system, preventive care currently includes blood tests and scanning procedures. Preventive care also seems to include the fear factor that sells many full body MRI procedures that are not only expensive but of dubious value[30].

Many blood tests are valuable in diagnosing life-threatening conditions. However, they sometimes lead to additional and unnecessary testing, stress and pain for the patient who ultimately is healthy and free of disease. This is considered to be preventive since it can be life saving.

Often, drugs are promoted and used in a preventive capacity for certain potential problems. For example, for years, doctors recommended their patients take an aspirin a day. Aspirin, a natural blood thinner, is recommended to decrease the likelihood of clots and therefore a benefit for both men and women.

Over the years, however, these recommendations were redefined and contra-indications have been spelled out. You can read the Mayo Clinic article at http://www.mayoclinic.com/health/daily-aspirin-therapy/HB00073, but the short of it is that aspirin does have side effects and it is important to be aware of them.

Be aware that seemingly innocent recommendations such as taking an aspirin-a-day include warnings to visit your doctor regularly to make sure this preventive regimen is not causing problems for you.

Other preventive measures taken by the health care system such as PSA tests, regular blood tests, breast exams, mammograms can save lives.

Nevertheless, sometimes these tests lead to invasive interventions that are not necessary. A recent example of this is the PSA test, used as a standard for diagnosing possible prostate cancer, which in older populations is slow growing due to its dependence on hormones.

A recent recommendation was to eliminate these screenings on men over 75 because it is of dubious value. Many older men had been subjected to procedures, some disabling, to correct a perceived threat that wasn't really there[31].

If these types of tests lead to other 'recommended' health procedural or diagnostic interventions, interview your doctor carefully. Do not let the fear factor take its toll on your psyche and make rash decisions resulting in an intervention that may not be necessary.

For example, there are vast numbers of women who unnecessarily opted for a double mastectomy as a preventive measure due to a family profile; or the removal of ovaries because of the fear of breast and ovarian cancer[32].

Of course, these drastic procedures are considered preventive, but they are also invasive and life altering and the effects can be far reaching including early menopause and body disfigurement.

Does The Benefit Outweigh The Risks?

Benefit-risk analysis should be the norm before agreeing to any intervention recommendation you receive from any health care provider.

What is the difference between an intervention and something that is preventive?

As mentioned previously, an example of preventive is a visit to your dentist who thoroughly cleans your teeth to prevent gum problems. Time and statistics have shown that this preventive procedure helps many people avoid gum disease and keep their original teeth instead of resorting to dentures as they age.

Yearly blood tests are interventional because they can lead to medications and other diagnostics that can have helpful effects but also if the tests are inaccurate, can lead to unneeded further interventions and procedures.

Cardiac stress tests are interventional too because their purpose is to determine if we need to do a significant life saving procedure, often in the absence of symptoms. They are also considered preventive because some people have heart problems and are not aware that their loss of energy or other vague symptoms are more serious. These screenings can save lives.

Knowing that your body type tends to tighten over time, it makes sense to schedule periodic visits to a qualified musculoskeletal specialist like a chiropractor to prevent the area from becoming so tight that it begins to affect the way you walk, affect the kinetic chain and create pain.

During a typical preventative visit, if a patient is tightening up, I loosen the appropriate muscles, and restore mobility to the area with a chiropractic adjustment which improves joint function. In the vast majority of cases, the patient leaves without experiencing the pain of a developing problem he did not even know is present.

Periodically, a patient is already in the process of becoming tight and walks with an irregular gait such as a limp. Observation dictates that it is then appropriate to recommend that he or she schedules a few visits to restore normal body mechanics.

The point is that these recommendations are low risk. Other than mild joint or muscle soreness as a side effect, the procedures are safe and prevent a problem that if not managed could instead require a many visits to resolve.

Interventional care can prevent pain and problems. It can save lives. It can also create an undesired consequence for someone who does not really have a problem... Do you know anyone burdened with a misinterpreted test result and over-reacting physicians?

Prevention should be about keeping you functioning at your best without invasive intervention; and, prevention has a lot to do with both lifestyle *and* body style.

When you, as a patient come to me in pain, I go through an extensive checklist. At the top of the list is:

- Do you have symmetry?
- Do you have other areas tightening that can eventually lead to a painful episode?
- Do you have another problem at which your primary care doctor should look?
- Do your symptoms and your patterns of dysfunction make sense functionally, or is there a more serious problem that requires further diagnostics?

Food for Thought...

Preventing health problems created by the American lifestyle is a full time job and obsession of mine. I regularly educate patients about the impact of diet on health and well-being.

In the U.S., most of us take in too many complex carbohydrates- those carbohydrates that the body breaks down into sugars[32]. A sedentary lifestyle and poor dietary practices unnecessarily creates more diabetics every day. We are not alone, though. Many countries that eat as we do exhibit otherwise preventative health problems found in the United States; problems such as heart disease and blood pressure.

In developed nations, over the years, the portions we eat became larger and many of the foods became unhealthy, laden with salt, and fat[33]. A purely preventive action is to decrease breads and complex carbohydrates and increase protein intake such as fish and meat. Do you remember the Atkins diet? High Protein, few carbohydrates. Simple.

Although many food experts criticize the Atkins' method, the experts do not dispute the many health benefits including lower insulin levels, lower weight and less food cravings. Many people on the Atkins diet see and feel these benefits[34].

Other studies suggest a modified Atkins diet that is not as carbohydrate restrictive to help solve a weight issue and the problems that eventually effect other body systems, joints and circulation of blood in the body.

You can read more about the benefits of a lower carbohydrate diet online at http://www.lowcarb.ca/articlesb/article338.html.

Do Your Feet "Stink?"

Scoliosis screening is required in schools. It makes sense. Checking for scoliosis is both preventive and can lead to intervention if it progresses. Consider the role your child's body asymmetry and foot overpronation has in his or her body development.

Overpronation can ultimately cause the rib cage to rotate creating idiopathic scoliosis (a curvature of the spine created by unknown causes) in portions of the population.

Twenty plus years of clinical experience leads me to the strong suspicion that overpronation with body asymmetry plays a major part of the development of idiopathic scoliosis. Nurses and other medical paraprofessionals often do scoliosis screenings in schools. It only takes another 20-30 seconds to check your child's feet.

Checking your child's feet as he or she develops and recommending shoe inserts to help prevent the debilitating experience of neck, back, knee, hip shoulder and other gait and asymmetry-related problems and preserve their knees is a purely quick, safe, and totally non-invasive preventive measure that gets results.

Overpronation:

According to Runners World Magazine, "it is the excessive inward roll of the foot after landing, such that the foot continues to roll when it should be pushing off. This twists the foot, shin and knee and can cause pain in all those areas (http://www.runnersworld.com/article/0%2C7120%2Cs6-240-319-327-425-0%2C00.html)."

This also creates a functional short leg, causing the surrounding muscles in the hip and abdomen to tighten, causing body asymmetry.

Idiopathic Scoliosis – Second Guessing the Condition

Common literature defines Scoliosis as a painful medical condition in which a person's spine curves abnormally from side to side in an "s" shape and can also be rotated. You can see this quite clearly on an x-ray.

Scoliosis typically has three classifications: congenital (anomalies in the vertebrae present at birth), idiopathic (meaning the condition develops at some point and sub-classified as infantile, juvenile, adolescent, or adult according to when onset occurs), or as a secondary symptom due to a physical trauma or from another condition such as cerebral palsy or spinal muscular atrophy.

Chapter sources include but are not limited to:

- http://www.wikipedia.org,
- http://adam.about.com/reports/Scoliosis.htm
- http://www.google.com/health,
- http://www.mayoclinic.com

Millions suffer from Idiopathic Scoliosis without having Cerebral Palsy, Muscular Atrophy, and physical trauma or because of abnormal vertebrae at birth. When we do not understand the cause, we use the term idiopathic. I first became very interested in idiopathic scoliosis while in school. If you have not already guessed, let me tell you that I do not like symptoms and conditions that do not have coherent explanations as to why they exist.

Scoliosis affects about 6 million people in the United States. The condition tends to run in families with people who have relatives with the condition having a 20% chance of developing the condition themselves. Until recently, medical science had no idea why or how scoliosis occurred. Then, in 2007, a ten-year study was published identifying the CHD7 gene in relationship to idiopathic scoliosis (representing 80% of all scoliosis patients). However, it is still unknown how this gene abnormality affects a person's chances of developing scoliosis.

Still, this gives a nudge in the right direction. There is now some serious thought being given to the idea that idiopathic scoliosis may be due to a wide variety of poorly understood inherited factors, most likely from the mother's side. However, the degree of severity can vary widely among family members with the condition, suggesting other factors may be present. I will address both the inherited factor and "other" factors in a moment.

It is public policy in schools across the country to screen students for Scoliosis, which, if the curve becomes too great, can be life threatening. Many of these children undergo screening during their annual physical. The test is simple, taking just seconds. The pediatrician has the child bend forward into what is called the Adams Position to see if the ribs create a hump on one side or the other, which is a prime diagnostic sign of the condition. If the hump is seen, a full spine x-ray is taken to determine the extent of the curve. We then wait, monitoring the curve to see if the condition progresses which is the typical medical protocol. Eventually, if the problem progresses sufficiently, medically, bracing is recommended and, in the worst cases, surgery using a Harrington rod to straighten the spinal curve.

However, why does this type of deformity really occur in the first place in seemingly normal developing bodies? Moreover, why is it more common in females (other than the obvious hormonal changes, females have a different body style than males, including a varying degree of wider hips depending on how their frame develops)?

I can definitively state that every case of Scoliosis I have ever treated has one thing in common. Every single Scoliosis patient I treat is built asymmetrically with an asymmetrical stance with most having moderate to severe overpronation, flat feet and foot flare.

Charschan's Working Theory on Idiopathic Scoliosis

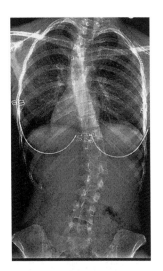

Idiopathic Scoliosis begins with gait asymmetry. It is likely that a child diagnosed with Idiopathic Scoliosis has never had his or her feet and gait evaluated because we do not evaluate for this because it is not public policy to do so.

The army routinely does this and has a protocol (army regulation 40-501) which has a solid rationale defined in the Army Standards of Medical Fitness Manual (mentioned earlier in this book)[35].

It is my medical opinion that we need to evaluate both feet and scoliosis while we are screening these children in school. This addition to the screening would not require additional time. I also firmly believe the mechanism of spinal curve development is describable as follows:

1. Child inherits significant gait asymmetry, likely with flat feet.
2. As young as 5-6 years, one side of the body is tighter than the other side. The child experiences growing pains as the body's bones fight to grow against muscles that are under excess tension already due to body asymmetry. (Often dismissed by pediatricians as something the child will grow out of as a normal part of body growth and maturation.)
3. Over time, the pelvis and lower back muscles begin to distort because of the way the child stands naturally, and the myofascia (the body connective tissue) reinforces torsion of the pelvis. The child will likely have flexibility problems, an important clue.

4. The psoas, the main hip flexor, will experience increased tension as the pelvis distorts. A distorted pelvis has little mechanical advantage and causes the muscles surrounding it to overcompensate and work harder to support the structure, while forcing the structure to recruit in other structures such as the legs and the upper body structures. The response is less flexibility and in many cases, abnormal motion and pain.

5. Over time, the tension on the anterior spine in the lower back from the psoas and its surrounding myofascia will increase, causing rotation of the developing segments in the spine and compensation in the motion segments above it.

6. As the child continues to grow, the distortion may become worse due to the continued tension (purely dependent on the degree of asymmetry and speed of growth). The more the child accommodates to the distortion, the more the myofascia surrounding the core muscles will enforce the curvature (perhaps, this is why curves even with bracing may continue to get progress).

7. As the distortion worsens, the bones form into the shape of the curve based on Wolf's law, a theory developed by the German Anatomist/Surgeon Julius Wolff in the mid-1800s that bone in a healthy person (or animal) adapts to the load under which it is placed (courtesy of wikipedia). This effect solidifies the permanency of the curve since distorted joints will yield permanently distorted structures.

8. Females are likely more affected because asymmetry has a greater effect on them due to their anatomic differences that may include wider hips, which will amplify problems that begin at the feet. (Could this also be why more females are classified with Fibromyalgia?).

9. When skeletal maturity is reached, the process slows markedly, although there are reports of slow continued progression throughout adulthood.

This model has yet to be proven clinically in studies outside my practice since I do not typically see children during school-screening years except as part of a sports injury assessment. However, since people who develop scoliosis may progress to a life-threatening curve, and since they are built asymmetrically and typically have flat feet, this relationship should taken more seriously and evaluated more thoroughly by screening children's feet when we evaluate them for curve progression. This, by definition, is a purely preventive health care screen that can help developing bodies without any harmful side effects if done correctly.

With 6 million people suffering, we need to reconsider the idea of watching and waiting and instead begin to look immediately at the body mechanically. Instead of managing curve progression, physicians need to understand the mechanics of the body better so that they can better predict who is at risk to develop Idiopathic Scoliosis and be better prepared with preventive and proactive solutions.

There needs to be more open discussion among providers of different disciplines regarding Idiopathic Scoliosis in order to arrive at an improved understanding of the condition and how to prevent it. Complimentary providers such as chiropractors have managed and in many cases, succeeded in reducing developing curves, thereby preventing the need to consider bracing or surgery. Methods such as these require further investigation[81].

It does not mean anything to treat something your specific medical discipline cannot understand within its current limited paradigm. There must be more openness between different mainstream and complimentary health care providers.

In our current system, we define idiopathic scoliosis but do not understand what causes the condition. We treat it as a disease instead of a manifestation of poor function. At best, ignoring function is wrong. At worst, it makes the medical community part of the problem.

Look at it this way. If you plant and grow a tree and apply forces to it, doing the same thing to it as our muscles potentially can do to a developing spine in response to asymmetry, the tree would also develop an irreversible curve as the bark and wood harden.

Upon identification of the potential for developing scoliosis based on the definitions I outlined, rather than just x-ray, sit and wait, an early alternative treatment following my medical practice patient experiences should include the following:

1. Off the shelf inserts for children that have gait asymmetries and flat feet that flare out. The benefits outweigh any risks.

2. Myofascial Release to core muscle and leg muscles to undo the effects of the asymmetrical forces on the spine before the curve progresses. If we find the problem early enough, we can react with treatment to change the tightness of the myofascia to allow better core stability, and potentially a better spinal adaptation pattern. Manipulation has proven helpful in the management of developing spinal curvatures[81].

3. Core strength and stabilization regimens are very important. Core muscles that distort the pelvis have little advantage against gravity, which tightens the upper back and leg muscles with the result being increased stress on the spinal, rib and extremity structures. The outcome is pain.

4. Monitor progression or regression of the curve with periodic plain film x-ray .

5. Referral to an pediatric orthopedic provider if curve continues progression past
25 degrees and shows no sign of resolution or regression.

Based on my experience implementing these types of regimens, an enlightened health care practitioner may ultimately reduce the need for bracing, corrective surgeries and reduce the number of adolescents living with significant curvatures that exist because we did not understand this condition well enough.

Notice, this protocol is active rather than passive. It includes referral if the problem does not resolve. This type of regimen potentially reduces problems, costs and pain with suffering since it performs early intervention and can markedly improve outcomes earlier.

Compare this to watch and wait. There is no contest.

Take Plantar Fasciitis... Please

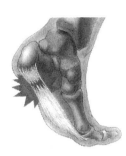

Doctors constantly compartmentalize different conditions; so the foot is looked at as if it is separate from the knee when it hurts, just as the knee is viewed as having no relationship to the structures above it. One example comes from the Medline e-letter. Medline is generally an informative web site for doctors. This e-letter referred to a study from the 2007 journal, Emergency Medicine, about Plantar Fasciitis:

Plantar Fasciitis: Evidence-Based Management

Plantar fascitis is the most common cause of a heel pain in adults and often one of the most frustrating. This evidence-based review explores etiology, management, and treatment.
-Medscape Emergency Medicine 2007

The article goes on and on about how to manage plantar fasciitis and how frustrating it is for both the doctor and the patient. Although the article is informative, breaking down the evidence it cites in the literature, the treatment is a dartboard approach of throwing therapies at the problem to see what works.

There is no observation or evidence cited that the people in the study have a harder heel strike (pounding the heel into the ground when we walk or run).

The article expresses little or no understanding of the mechanism behind the hard heel strike. It just states what the name of the condition is, how it involves the local area that exhibits the symptoms and offers multiple therapies to try when somebody has these symptoms.

They should have asked me, or asked someone like me. In my experience, plantar fasciitis results from a heavy heel strike secondary to overpronation that begins in the feet, affects the pelvis, which tightens the legs and affects the way you walk.

Even though the current literature supports the idea that if the core muscles are firing poorly the legs will tighten and cause a heavy heel strike, there is no mention of poor muscle firing patterns relationship to plantar fasciitis in this particular paper. The article follows the typical pattern we see in diagnosis and treatment of conditions rather than addressing the functional mechanical cause, something that is quite apparent when you place the patient on a treadmill, as you will clearly hear banging upon heel strike. By the way, many running stores now have treadmills, allowing you to see this on yourself in slow motion. If you have this condition, this is a great way to self diagnose!

The study recommendations for treatment include a list of widely accepted treatments to the area or pain, rather than to the gait issue creating it, in the hope that something will work:

- Achilles Tendon Stretching
- Rest
- Taping
- Night Splints
- Heel Pads and Orthotics
- Extracorporeal Shock-Wave Therapy
- Surgery

The study summarizes findings of what the condition is:
- Plantar fascitis is an injury of overuse and is unrelated to trauma.
- The condition is due to micro tears in the collagen fibers of the plantar fascia.

- Plantar fascitis represents a tendonosis, not an inflammatory condition.
- Symptoms are due to fascial strain at the take-off phase of walking, not heel impact.
- Clinicians should look for alternative causes of pain in adolescent and elderly patients.
- The diagnosis is a clinical one in the majority of cases. Radiographs are of limited value.
- Up to 85% of patients will improve independent of the mode of therapy used, if at all.

There is little mention about body mechanics. All the information limited to the feet. It promotes the myth of overuse. Millions of people walk long distances yet only certain people with certain body mechanical styles are prone to plantar fasciitis.

Sure, micro-tears in the collagen fibers exist but again, why does this develop on certain people and not others? The reason of course, is that you must look at the body to get the answer, not just the foot. Since all treatment they recommend is toward the symptomatic part, not toward the malfunction, clinicians who use this information neither truly understand this condition nor can treat it effectively on a consistent enough basis. Meanwhile, the patient is stuck in a hamster wheel stressing the plantar fascia and continually re-injuring the part or experiencing problems in other parts of the kinetic chain such as knee, hip or back pain.

The article gives the following problem management pearls:
- Allow an adequate trial of rest and stretching before instituting more aggressive or invasive therapies.
- Corticosteroids increase the risk of rupture of the plantar fascia and provide only short-term relief in most cases.
- The evidence for use of non-custom-made orthotics, night splints, or heel pads is minimal.
- ESWT (Extracorporeal Shock Wave Therapy) may be considered prior to resorting to a surgical approach. Its use is controversial, and there are conflicting reports in the literature[36].

- Consider surgery as the last option for patients who fail to respond to conservative measures.

While all this is probably within reason to most physicians who were to think this way, the problem is never explained from a mechanical standpoint detailing the true role of gait (the way we walk) in creating the condition. The recommended treatments are clearly hit or miss and based solely on symptoms, not on function.

Because the article explains in detail what the condition "is thought" to be by its authors and what happens in the tissues we are supposed to assume we know what we are treating. The real problem here, the condition in the tissues, is merely the tip of the iceberg and plantar fasciitis is merely a result of the way the person has adapted to their body style.

Seriously, if plantar fasciitis was simply due to foot overuse, wouldn't everyone experience it? Why doesn't staying off it allow you to feel better until you begin running again or until you grow tolerant of pain on the bottom of your foot?

There exists a huge knowledge gap here.

How does the condition occur and why? If your health care provider does not understand how and why the condition occurs, how can he understand what he is treating? Simply, he cannot, which leads down the path of treating the symptom and not the problem- which is gait- and is passed on within families.

It is well established that we pass body features from generation to generation. Shouldn't your health practitioner know and consider this. Your practitioner and you should   look at your family tree and see how many people have or had problems like those you experience from time to time. Are the problems you experience during your life happenstance or destiny?

The Value and Cost of Emergency Care

There are many good ideas in the current American health care system; especially when it comes to emergency medicine that proves helpful in life threatening situations.

The U.S. has some of the finest emergency medicine centers in the world. However, many non life-threatening problems are treated and diagnosed as if they are life threatening disease states. The result is huge health care costs, and great emotional cost to the person experiencing the problem and his or her family. The truth is that many of these costs can be avoided with better and more complete evaluations of the musculoskeletal system to guide the person to a better diagnosis, leading to effective treatment options rather than additional expensive tests.

? ? ? could be better worded - - -

Only a crazy person would argue against a sensible evaluation and treatment. Only a total nutcase would argue against a need for a more reasonable cost structure to health care evaluation, testing and treatment.

A while ago my son went to the hospital for a gash in his hand. He required about 10 stitches. The visit lasted an hour and the bill was for just under $1000 dollars. Why should sewing human skin cost so much? What is the cost of the materials? What is the cost of the facility? What is the true cost?

A patient of mine is an emergency room (ER) doctor who works at a walk-in clinic run by doctors who formerly worked in hospital ERs. Few people I know consider going to a walk-in clinic for the kind of wound my son had, probably because most people just don't know that they can. However, this former ER doctor said her facility charges under $300 for the type of evaluation and stitching service my son required.

Ouch! This seems to be a huge argument for the U.S. to finally devise a sensible health care system vs. the current system which is often premium priced when compared to costs in other countries with similar economies. The potential savings could likely insure everyone in the country.

Of course, the larger issue is that more 'expensive care' does not necessarily make 'better care'. While everyone wants to come to the U.S. to learn how to be a doctor, the U.S. is not high on the lists of health care systems compared to other countries that cover their populations effectively from cradle to grave. Perhaps we need better transparency, so the public can compare the prices for services, which may in effect drive down prices for many medical services.

Squeezing Out Providers

Over time, the health care system has squeezed out many legitimate competing health care providers and health care provider groups.

When is the last time you heard of, or sought out the help of a naprapath? **Naprapathy** focuses on healing methods that work through the connective tissues that hold your skeleton together. Connective tissues include ligaments, tendons, and muscles that are flexible and resilient when you are healthy. In a way, a naprapath is a lot like a chiropractor for soft tissue.

How about a naturopath? **Naturopathy** emphasizes natural remedies like a healthy diet and exercise to heal the body rather than surgery or synthetic drugs.

Others, like the osteopath, successfully assimilated into the current health care system and are very often your primary care doctor. A few even perform manipulation (like a chiropractor).

However, as my own primary doctor (an osteopath) freely admits, the insurance companies either pay you as a primary doctor or as a specialist doctor who provides manipulation thereby creating a disincentive for primary physicians to perform manipulation, which in turn could contain some costs.

He told me, "I would rather send a patient who needs manipulation to you."

What Else Can Go Wrong?

Insurance companies created an entirely new category of unnecessary medical expense by refusing to pay doctors to visit their patients during rounds in the hospital. Do you know who is just as likely now to see you while you are laid up in the hospital bed? A hospitalist. These are doctors who visits you instead of your doctor, and reports to your doctor on your condition. They typically charge higher fees than what your doctor did years ago before insurance companies stopped paying doctors to visit their patients in the hospital.

This is just one more of the many cost drivers in a system that the insurance companies have created by underpaying your primary doctor. It is time our country makes the hard decisions and reinvents health care for the people it serves, rather than for the sustainability of our currently expensive and not necessarily more effective system.

As I am writing this book, I have read many articles about how we have to pay for our new system. To silence the detractors of a single payer government run system, the insurance companies, American Medical Association, and American Hospital Association who all stand to either gain or lose by appropriately changing our current system volunteered to reduce health cost increases by 1 ½ percent.

They claim this will be a significant cost savings over time. Unfortunately, much of what we do is probably not adding to our long-term survival. If, however, we reform health care properly, and embrace a wellness model rather than our current sickness model, costs can be substantially reduced, we will require fewer specialists, and there will be many types of primary care providers to choose from.

A legitimate overhaul likely includes medical schools shifting focus back to primary care because of primary care doctors being paid more, and specialists being revered less. Doctors will be less incentivized for doing many procedures, and more incentivized for better outcomes. The idea of the family doctor will become more important as your doctor can once again afford to spend time evaluating and listening to you, because he is now incentivized to do so.

When you have musculoskeletal complaints, future doctors will look at you, not just your symptoms. Finally, the system will likely cost substantially less than today with people requiring fewer drugs and replacement parts as we retain the joints in our bodies because they did not wear out. With a focus on prevention, our diets will likely get better; we will get more exercise and age more gracefully and enjoy a better quality of life.

> **"The way I look at this, we need to fundamentally change the relationship we have with the (health care) delivery system."**
>
> *July 23, 2010, New Jersey Star Ledger* quotes William J. Marina, 3.8 million member Horizon Blue Cross Blue Shield of New Jersey chairman, president and chief executive regarding a pilot program where family-practice doctors, cancer specialists, orthopedists and a pharmaceutical company will be paid for the quality care rather than the quantity of care.

This, of course, is a health care utopia. One can only hope.

SECTION II

Your Doctor

Health Care's Gatekeepers

Primary care providers are the gatekeepers to our health care system. Specifically, the primary care physician who handles only certain diagnostics in the office, coordinates your care during times of illness and refers you to other specialists in the medical system as he (or she) deems appropriate.

In our health care system, gatekeepers are usually either Medical Doctors (MD) or Doctors of Osteopathy (DO) providers. However, often patients instead see the Nurse Practitioner or Physicians Assistant, also known as physician extenders. Although uncommon, in medically underserved areas a different kind of first contact provider is known to assume the role of primary care provider... including the chiropractor.

Health Maintenance Organizations (HMO's) limit their pool of providers either by paying them poorly as compared to their out of network counterparts or by limiting the amount of specialists in a certain category. In theory, doctors would see more patients in exchange for discounted fees and more business.

HMO plans ration health care through the primary care provider who is responsible for referrals, known as the gatekeeper. For you, this means that based on his (or her) experience, training or personal and professional bias that your doctor determines whom you may or may not see.

To make ends meet, doctors modify their practices to see more people in less time, use physician extenders (nurse practitioners, physician's assistants) and to see more people at a lower cost, making your care in many offices less personal. The doctors staff handles referrals to specialist providers on your insurance companies list. Essentially, your doctor feeds the system.

Because of your doctor's medical training, he comes from a culture of the symptom and disease paradigm, rather than a functional one.

It is more common than you might want to think. Most medically based providers see symptoms from a disease and drug treatment point of view and commonly will refer to specialists based on the suspected body system or part (s) that may be problematic.

This is why if you have gastrointestinal distress, you are typically referred to a specialist who looks only at that system. If you suffer shoulder pain, you are referred to an orthopedist that specialized in the shoulder.

If you have knee pain, you see a specialist who looks just at the knee, and if you have back pain, you see a specialist who looks at the back.

If you have cancer, you see an oncologist.

You get the idea.

A patient recently told me that after a fall she had to visit three doctors to figure out her pain: one doctor for her knee who performed an MRI and other tests, a second doctor who looked at her ankle and a third for her back.

Her primary care doctor finally decided to recommend her to someone who would look at her as a person, instead of as several disconnected painful parts and symptoms that needed evaluation.

In my experience, it always makes sense to evaluate the mechanisms behind the symptom and not just the symptom. The ankle, knee, hip and lower back are part of an integrated movement system. Therefore, the patient should have had the entire leg and back evaluated during the initial visit, rather than just the knee.

It is a fact that health care costs escalate when your primary care doctor believes you need a referral. You begin to visit other medical specialists, endure tests and find yourself going from doctor to doctor looking for an answer that never seems to come.

It was different in 'the old days.' Years ago, most doctors looked at your symptoms but often treated you as a whole (holistically). They were capable and able to manage many more conditions without referring you to a specialist. Your doctor used to rely on his hands and diagnostic skills rather than expensive tests...

Do You Want Fries With That?

Unfortunately, there is also another developing problem to tackle. I call it 'Fast Food Medicine'.

There is a change occurring as mini-clinics with nurse practitioners open in CVS and Walmart with their Minute clinic (www.minuteclinic.com). However, they can only address a limited number of the most common conditions and come from the same disease, symptom treatment and drug paradigm.

The mini-clinics work off the basis that they are fast, convenient and relatively inexpensive when compared to a physician visit. Since many are located inside the drug store, they can prescribe the medication you require, thereby feeding the profits of the store pharmacy in which they are situated. The health care providers are physician extenders only, such as nurse practitioners. They work because those who believe they require a prescription can easily go to the clinic, and then walk across the store to their pharmacy where they receive their medication.

There is no question that this is convenient for the consumer. Since many of these clinics also have contracts with your insurance carrier, you may only have to pay your co-payment for the visit, making these clinics even more attractive as busy patient juggling the kids' schedules while working two jobs to pay the mortgage.

Disjointed Health care Training and Treatment

Ironically, when it comes to understanding how the skeletal system works, our health care system is horribly disjointed and broken.

clumzy wording

Over-specialization has created a symptom-based system of treating painful regions of the body as if the pain is the cause.

Sure, certain kinds of trauma require a specialist. However, pre-injury body mechanics typically are ignored when an injury occurs. The way a person is built may have predisposed them to the very injury being treated.

Body style and build is ignored when looking at joint damage that seems to have an obvious cause. Screening people for body style issues when they are younger can prevent many injuries to the skeletal system, especially as you age.

The symptom-disease and drug idea of managing the musculoskeletal system often leads to improper conclusions. This is because the area of symptom(s) is not necessarily the true problem that is creating the condition, and prescribing medication to reduce pain and inflammation for a condition your physician does not understand makes little sense.

The way we are built affects the way our body works. A great example of this is shoulder pain.

A patient visiting from another state was experiencing shoulder pain on her right side. Her orthopedic specialist evaluated her right shoulder and saw that it rolled forward and down and recommended she visit a physical therapist for a few visits. Luckily, she never made it to a physical therapist. She came to me first.

I evaluated her and found that her abdominal left oblique muscle (located to the left of her belly button) was shortened and tightened, preventing her from lifting her arm properly. My evaluation clearly showed the problem was in her lower back region, not her shoulder. The problem just symptomatically presented itself in her right shoulder.

Visually, I could see that her pelvis was torqued (distorted), however, she reported that as far as she could tell, her lower back was neither sore nor stiff. She did report that the muscles were tender in the lower back.

I treated her with Myofascial release to the muscles in the lower back, her abdominal area as well as her left hip muscles.

Once the muscles in her lower back, left oblique muscle and hip were treated using myofascial release treatment, her shoulder pain resolved and she had full pain-free range of motion at the conclusion of the visit. I then instructed her in postural upper body improvement exercises.

Had she previously completed the recommended month of physical therapy to 'treat' her painful shoulder, it is likely she would have further aggravated the situation because she would have been treating the symptom instead of the actual mechanical cause of her shoulder pain.

Because the shoulder was functioning poorly and was pulled forward, loading the joint further with exercises would have made the muscles tighter and eventually caused her to experience shoulder blade pain and neck pain as well.

> Many people experiencing disappearing pain in one area, relieved by treating another, are more than a little bit intrigued because it goes against everything they instinctually believe- that the painful part must be the problem.

This example illustrates the problem with our current paradigm that teaches health care providers and patients to look at the symptom as if it is a unique and discrete problem. There is commonly an underlying belief that a patient must have done something to create the current problem, and health care providers must attempt to apply a treatment to the painful area(s).

The Fibromyalgia Myth Factory and a $3 Million Dollar Reward

Unfortunately, when you have pain all over the body, like many people 'diagnosed' with Fibromyalgia (an attempt to group or classify Myofascial pain that is throughout the body), or other systemic problems, finding the right solution becomes even more frustrating.

You are forced to manage with a chronic pain you do not understand because given your doctor's diagnostic background he struggles to come up with a solution to a problem he cannot understand.

Add to your problem the lack of coordinating systems within the health care system. Diagnosing the problem can be herculean task with ever-increasing costs. Every doctor has his own database of patients resulting in many tests needlessly duplicated.

> I cannot stress the need to rethink our way of health care that is integrative not just by name, but by paradigm.

Based on more than two decades of experience treating people who have lived for years with chronic symptoms, our obsession with symptom diagnosis instead of functionally looking at the bigger picture, and understanding the systems that create pain and body breakdown has left many people searching for alternatives to the traditional health care approach of drugs, tests, exercises and surgeries.

Fibromyalgia and Myofascial Pain Syndromes

(Sources include but are not limited to: _www.webmd.com/fibromyalgia/default.htm; www.mayoclinic.com/health/ fibromyalgia/DS00079; www.wikipedia.org/wiki/Fibromyalgia.)*

Fibromyalgia (FM) is a disorder classified by the presence of chronic widespread pain and tactile allodynia (abnormal pain sensitivity). An example of tactile allodynia is a person who perceives light pressure or the movement of clothes over the skin as painful, whereas a healthy individual will not feel pain.

A number of symptoms other than pain often affecting Fibromyalgia patients, includes:
- debilitating fatigue,
- abnormal sleep architecture, meaning the brain does not reach all the restorative levels of sleep necessary for overall health,
- functional bowel disturbances and
- a variety of neuropsychiatric problems including cognitive dysfunction, which can mean short and long term memory problems, slowed information processing ability, diminished attention span and anxiety and depressive symptoms.

While the criteria for such an entity have not yet been thoroughly developed, the recognition that fibromyalgia involves more than just pain has led to the frequent use of the term "fibromyalgia syndrome."

It is not contagious. However, recent studies suggest that people with fibromyalgia may be genetically predisposed. Fibromyalgia affects more females than males, with a ratio of 9:1 by American College of Rheumatology (ACR) criteria.

Fibromyalgia affects about 2% of the general population and is most commonly diagnosed in individuals between the ages of 20 and 50, though onset can occur in childhood.

Are you ready for a surprise? After reading this far, you may expect me to argue there is no such thing as fibromyalgia. Here is the shock. Based on years of experience, I do think the condition exists. However, the diagnostic criteria used by the American College of Rheumatology (ACR) is suspect, since it allows many of these patients to be wrongly classified when they actually have a condition known as Myofascial Pain Syndrome.

Based on over 20 years in practice, I am convinced that many people who are in chronic pain are misunderstood and over-medicated because their physicians just do not understand how someone could be in chronic pain like this.

Labeling chronic pain throughout the body as Fibromyalgia allows doctors to use diagnostic criteria to classify this as a disease. The problem with this is that the condition usually has a functional basis in the majority of cases I have seen in practice.

> **myofascial**
> [m·fash·l]
>
> pertaining to a muscle and its sheath of connective tissue, or fascia.
>
> Source: Mosby's Medical Dictionary, 8th edition. © 2009, Elsevier.

While the medical community at large gives a slight nod to the idea of genetic predisposition, two things reinforce my belief that this painful condition is absolutely inherited.

First, biomechanical problems are passed from generation to generation (you not only look like them but walk like them too!); and second, "fibromyalgia" is more predominant in women. Women have wider hips and increase angles at the knees and other joints. Body asymmetry affects women more adversely than men.

Myofascial Pain Syndrome (or MPS) is a term used to describe one of the conditions characterized by chronic pain. It is associated with and caused by "trigger points" (TrPs), which are sensitive and painful areas between the muscle and fascia. The symptoms can range from referred pain through myofascial trigger points to specific pains in other areas of the body.

Fibromyalgia and Myofascial Pain Syndrome sound similar. As a patient, how can you know one condition from the other? Can your doctor tell the difference? Can you be sure of a proper diagnosis?

Fibromyalgia Diagnostic Criteria Versus Body Asymmetry

In studying the criteria of diagnosing fibromyalgia, it is important to note that there are many similarities to the Brian Rothbart model of bio-implosion referenced later in the book and the overall effect on the joints, ligaments and muscles and tendons in the musculoskeletal

> Dr. Rothbart teaches and practices pain elimination techniques. He currently resides and practices in Europe.
>
> You can learn more at www.rothbartsite.com

system. Of course, fibromyalgia uses a "Tender Point" scale for assessment.

A sensible argument, one I make after more than twenty years helping over 4,600 patients, is that the tender points that are diagnostic for Fibromyalgia are actually an expression of body asymmetry, bio-implosion and myofascial adaptation (also discussed in more detail later).

I further contend that the medical community has adapted these expressions of body asymmetry to fit the Fibromyalgia classification, which is really nothing more than a collection of symptoms and signs grouped together in an attempt to create an inclusive classification describing the phenomenon.

Fibromyalgia and Myofascial Pain Syndrome is an expression of poor body structure. If addressed early in life, it is likely we can prevent people from suffering from many chronic systemic pain syndromes that fall under the medical classification of Fibromyalgia.

The phenomenon of Fibromyalgia is still poorly misunderstood. In an attempt to classify why they are in pain, people are commonly mislabeled, subjected to ideas, treatments and medications that are of minimal value in helping them achieve a more normal and pain free existence. The Fibromyalgia classification is a strong argument for a functional diagnostic model versus the Fibromyalgia tender point classification tool.

The American College of Rheumatology (ACR) uses tender points as a means of classifying an individual as having fibromyalgia for both clinical and research purposes.

Below are the the classic Fibromyalgia diagnostic tender points and how they relate to the changes that occur from foot flare and bio-implosion.

1. The base of the skull beside the spinal column.
2. The base of the neck in the back.
3. The top of the shoulder toward the back.

4.   The breastbone.

5.   The outer edge of the forearm about 2 cm below the elbow.

6.   The shoulder blade.

7.   The top of the hip

8.   The outside of the hip.

9.   The fat pad over the knee.

During diagnosis, force (about the amount of pressure required to blanch the thumbnail when applying pressure) is exerted at each of the 18 points. The patient must feel pain at 11 or more of these points for fibromyalgia to be considered.

Additional criterion includes a history of widespread pain has been present for at least three months. Pain is considered widespread when the following are present:

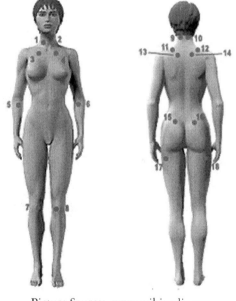

- Pain in both sides of the body.
- Pain above and below the waist.
- Axial skeletal pain (cervical spine, anterior chest, thoracic spine or low back pain must be present).
- Low back pain is considered lower segment pain.
- Interrupted sleep is common with this condition.

Picture Source: www.wikipedia.org

The following is a list of conditions and the percent diagnosed (or misdiagnosed) as symptoms of Fibromyalgia Syndrome. It is an attempt of the American College of Rheumatology (ACR) to classify musculoskeletal pain as a disease process.

Condition	% Diagnosed as Symptoms of FMS
Muscular Pain	100
Fatigue	96
Insomnia	86
Joint Pains	72
Headaches	60
Restless Legs	56
Numbness and Tingling	52
Impaired Memory	46
Leg Cramps	42
Impaired Concentration	41
Nervousness	32
Depression (Major Depression)	20

While the classification seems simple, the real question is, "What is a tender point and why is it tender?"

The criteria rely on tenderness in the classification but neither defines tenderness, nor explores why the part is tender. Color me crazy, but shouldn't it matter why the part is sore to the touch?

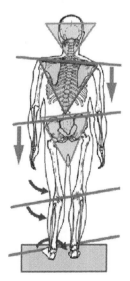

If you view this as a functional problem, joints under strain are tender to the touch. It then becomes important to ask why the joints are under strain; something that can only be answered by looking at the problem functionally.

Let us look at our model for asymmetry. People with asymmetry and gait issues secondary to kinetic chain dysfunction present like this as well. Is it possible the ACR is attempting to describe people with gait issues that result in body wide pain without realizing it? Is it possible that the ACR's thought process, which is symptomatic and not structural, is missing the point?

So which is it? Does body asymmetry equal Fibromyalgia or Myofascial Pain Syndrome? Let us bust a couple of myths and open up some alternative possibilities...

Patients who overpronate and are asymmetrical in their build will also have tenderness in the following areas (working up from the feet):

Fibromyalgia diagnostic tender point #9; The fat pad over the knee.

When you overpronate with foot flare, you also have internal rotation of the tibia (shin bone) when you walk with each step. If bad enough, this will eventually create knock knee's as you wear down the medial meniscus in the knee (one of the cushions in the knee) over time from excess wear and tear due to the knee rolling in too much as you walk. This is inappropriately called overuse rather than a consequence of body style. The result is that the fat pad (the tissue on medial side of your knee) bulges on the inside of the knee and becomes tender. Fibromyalgia diagnostic tender point #9; The fat pad over the knee... **Busted.**

Fibromyalgia diagnostic tender point #8; The outside of the hip.

When the tibia (the shin bone) rotates in, so does the femur (the upper leg bone) during overpronation. The result is increased stress in the tissues on the lateral leg by the hip as described in the criteria. These tissues will become thickened and painful over time, becoming a source of chronic pain for many people. Fibromyalgia diagnostic tender point #8; The outside of the hip... **Busted.**

Fibromyalgia diagnostic tender point #7; The top of the hip.

The hip drops, which, over time, makes the top of the hipbones (the inominate) tender from the gluteal muscles in the buttock tightening at their insertion points. The hip drop and tightened gluteal muscles causes the body to accommodate with the shortening and tightening of the latissimus dorsi insertions and the erector spinae insertions (both insert into the lower back into the area of the inominate). Typically, this tender point presents in people whose frames have a significant amount of asymmetry which torques the pelvis (tortipelvis) creating poor movement coordination, resulting in muscle shortening, tightening and poor movement coordination. Fibromyalgia diagnostic tender point #7; The top of the hip... **Busted**.

Fibromyalgia diagnostic tender point #4; The shoulder blade, breastbone and clavicle.

Typically, when the foot turns out, the body leans the rib cage forward on the same side in compensation. The psoas muscle and the core muscles (the rectus abdominus and oblique muscles) tighten in response to foot asymmetry. When this change in posture occurs, the posterior muscles in the shoulder blade tighten because the change in the angle at which the shoulder works altering the firing pattern, causing strain as the rib cage is rotated on the opposite side. The net effect is chronic tightness in the shoulders blades, reduced range of motion in the neck, and problems in the arms. As the ribs rotate, their insertions become tender at the front and the chest will have tender areas along the breast bone where they insert. The shoulder blades will be especially tight and tender on the side of rotation and the clavicle insertions will be sore because the rotation of the rib cage strains their insertions. Fibromyalgia diagnostic tender point #4; Tenderness of the shoulder blade, breastbone and clavicle... **Busted**.

Fibromyalgia diagnostic tender point #5; The outer edge of the forearm about 2 cm below the elbow.

When the shoulder leans forward, it results in reduced external rotation in the shoulder, which causes strain at the elbow. The muscles then tighten creating soreness at the outer edge of the forearm. Fibromyalgia diagnostic tender point #5; The outer edge of the forearm about 2 cm below the elbow... **Busted**.

Fibromyalgia diagnostic tender point #6; The top of the shoulder toward the back.

As the shoulders are pulled forward, the posterior shoulder muscles become tight into the levator scapula and upper traps. This is exacerbated by muscular recruitment (using other muscles in that area to help resulting from poorly coordinated movement) into this region when we use the shoulder because of the angle of pull these muscles have about a poorly positioned joint. Fibromyalgia diagnostic tender point #6; The top of the shoulder toward the back... **Busted**.

Fibromyalgia diagnostic tender points #1, #2, and #3; The base of the skull beside the spinal column and the base of the neck in the back.

When the changes discussed in diagnostic points 4, 5, 6, 7, 8 and 9 happen, the muscular insertions at the upper neck become tender due to recruitment of the levator scapula with shoulder joint activities, which uses the muscle improperly when it rolls forward. As the levator scapula shortens over time and becomes tighter the effect is increased tension at the base of the skull. The tight muscles alter upper neck motion, as well as develop scar tissue at insertions in both the scapula and skull, which become sources of chronic tenderness as well as triggers for headaches as the tight muscle's lack of elasticity irritates the upper spinal segments in the neck by the base of the skull. Also involved are the posterior scalene muscles and upper trapezious, which insert along the spinal segments in the neck and cause chronic soreness and pain. Fibromyalgia diagnostic tender points #1, #2, and #3; The base of the skull beside the spinal column and the base of the neck in the back...
Busted.

It is not a coincidence that tender points mirror Dr. Rothbart's bio-implosion model. The resulting strain renders the stress points tender to the touch. Tender points have a functional basis. Using non-functional criteria solely due to tenderness

> The Fibromyalgia diagnostic criteria are a static, non-functional model.

from a certain amount of pressure is somewhat meaningless. Other than the soreness at the point of contact, the health care provider will have no idea why the area is sore. He only knows that it is sore, and that "fact" can be used to classify a person with chronic pain as a "Fibromyalgia sufferer". This does little to help the health care provider find an effective therapeutic method since function is not considered, and, as you just read, tender points appear to be a side effect of poor function.

The Fibromyalgia disease classification attempts to create criteria for physicians to group people with common tender points, sleep deprivation and pain sensitivity that the ACR cannot explain using the current static model. The problem is that it leaves health care providers clueless as to how to go about finding an answer to a patient's problem. That is why people who truly have problems with pain regulation often get confused with people with functional pain.

In my years of experience, very few patients labeled with the term Fibromyalgia actually have pain levels that are way out of proportion to what their practitioner finds during an evaluation. Most people with true Fibromyalgia (when the pain is out of proportion to what is found and varies from day to day without any consistency) are far and few between.

People classified with Fibromyalgia are given medications such as anti-depressants, and are told to exercise (although ill advised if their bodies are not functioning well mechanically) because the endorphin release during their exercise regimen gives them some pain relief. [37] Studies show that people with Fibromyalgia Syndrome find regular exercise helps lessen the pain. [38] In those who run, endorphins are thought to be responsible for the effect called the "runners high."

Not so long ago it was theorized that intolerance to one's own thyroxin (thyroid hormone) was the cause of Fibromyalgia. However, when the test patients were tested, they had normal levels of the hormone. Interestingly, although the patients had normal levels of the hormone, some patients experienced a reduction of symptoms when receiving thyroid supplementation medication.[39] Of course, it may just have been a placebo-effect reaction. These studies were published in the now out-of-print "Clinical Bulletin of Myofascial Therapy."

Other studies focus on anti-depressant therapy as helpful in treating "Fibromyalgia" patients.[40]

Unfortunately, in the absence of an evaluation, that researches the structural, chemical and mechanical together in a cohesive evaluation method that makes sense, the diagnosis of Fibromyalgia is common. When a person has chronic widespread myofascial pain that defies the understanding of your health care provider, he looks for a coherent treatment method. He tries to fit your symptoms into the criteria from the board of Rheumatology because it is widely accepted by the medical profession as a disease process.

Instead, your doctor should be looking at function and your body style because, as you will come to understand from this book, this type of pain and inherited body style issues are inseparable.

The currently accepted research and definitions of Fibromyalgia and Myofascial Pain Syndrome suggest there is evidence showing a genetic predisposition (body style inherited). Women are more prone to acquire the condition, which may again imply body style issues. Women with wide hips have an increased angle of pull at the knees and ankles. Women built more asymmetrically tend to experience more pain because the wider hips and accommodation at the knees and ankles amplify the effect of overpronation when compared to the build of a comparable male or woman with narrower hips.

Specialists, (e.g. rheumatologist) for chronic inflammatory disease processes evaluate many people suffering chronic pain throughout the body even though it is more appropriate and cost effective to evaluate them from a functional basis first. A very small portion of the populace has Lupus, Rheumatoid Arthritis and other chronic systemic body disease processes. The rest of the populace is suffering from chronic musculoskeletal problems misunderstood because of our obsession with symptoms, rare diseases and our misunderstanding of function as it relates to those symptoms at an incredible cost to society. It is not an exaggeration. Just read your favorite news website or newspaper...

> # Jury awards woman $3M for pain linked to minor crash
>
> by Sue Epstein, Star-Ledger Staff
>
> The August 25, 2010 New Jersey Star Ledger reported a jury deliberated and awarded $3 Million dollar settlement to a Manalapan woman claiming widespread body pain as a result of a minor fender-bender that caused no damage to either car, nor obvious damage to either driver. She walked away from the accident feeling fine, and developed pain symptoms twelve hours later. She sought the help of specialists in the following months, each providing a slightly different diagnosis, until it was "determined" the cause of her pain was neurologically induced from the trauma from the minor auto accident. Several expert witness physicians testified the woman has CRSD- complex regional pain syndrome, causing debilitating pain in her neck and back.
>
> The woman received daily infusions of ketamine (an anesthetic) for two weeks, with eight boosters since the initial treatment; and her doctors want to increase the dosage.
>
> The defense argued, and lost, that she does not have CRSD, but instead suffers from non-related Fibromyalgia.

With so many doctors looking at the woman, I am sure the woman is suffering pain. Unfortunately, no one has looked at her functionally and definitively identified the cause of her pain except to say it was the fault of the accident and deserves a multi-million dollar payday when the car incident may have simply brought an existing problem to light exacerbated by the minor trauma. This is exactly the kind of patient who needs to seek out a different kind of doctor, rather than the symptom-disease trained specialists who are relegating her to a life of injections to feel "a little bit better."

Of course, the primary goal is to get the patient healthy again. However, I am just as sure the defense attorney and insurance company would be interested in a functional diagnosis. One that is easier for patient, judge and jury to understand.

Understanding the mechanics behind Myofascial Pain Syndrome/ Fibromyalgia can lead to improved diagnosis and treatment based on improvement of function and symmetry as opposed to the ACR criteria of tender points, which clearly are not understood other than that they have been consistently observed.

Observation by a health care provider without a clear understanding of causation is of little help to patient's search for effective treatments. It is more a source of frustration for anyone going through the current health care system wondering why nobody understands why he or she is in pain.

Current studies show an increasing population is embracing alternative and complimentary health care providers to get relief beyond what the traditional health care systems paradigm is capable of offering. [41]

Back pain, neck pain, shoulder problems and many other painful conditions in the musculoskeletal system often fail to respond to 'traditional' medical treatment because traditional health care medical schools teach health care providers that each condition is its own entity, rather than teaching doctors to understand that the pain it is a result of a poor functioning system or systems.

Insurance company coding reinforces this line of thinking since every symptom must have a code. However, the codes typically describe the symptomatic part rather than the dysfunction that is causing the area to become symptomatic. Directing a trial of care based on a symptomatic region is common accepted practice. Patients have learned to expect this as well, since they have grown up with a system that closely relates symptoms to the problem, when in fact, in the musculoskeletal system, the true cause is often not at the site of symptoms.

Fixing this problem requires we must change the way doctors understand, evaluate and ultimately treat back pain and other conditions involving the spine and its affiliated structures that include the arms and legs.

The belief that you can break down the body into different organs and joints and then specialize in the treatment of the parts instead of the whole is very simply inefficient, expensive and leaves patients with uncured problems even after investing time, effort and money investigating alternatives after the traditional model has not solved their problem satisfactorily.

This has led to the steady rise of alternative or complimentary care providers who have a different thought process. Solutions that have higher patient satisfaction exist in the growing industry of complementary medicine. Patient satisfaction has been shown to be high and people are increasingly willing to pay for it even when their insurance company will not cover this type of care.

The musculoskeletal, hormonal and neurological systems of the body have interconnected pathways. Since systems of the body function interdependently, some in ways we have yet to fully understand, having specialists trained to see the symptoms as if they are the problem is often the problem.

Moreover, this 'traditional' diagnostic way of thinking is a major reason we see deteriorating health and escalating health care costs as people age.

The Scientific Myths of Back and Neck Pain Treatment

OR "Deductive reasoning with rational treatment" Vs. "Name it and hope the therapy we are using works."

A case can now be made that conditions such as neck pain, shoulder pain, sciatica pain, and hip pain actually come from the same mechanical source.

Most health care providers are taught to believe that the area of symptoms is the cause of the conditions in the musculoskeletal system. They are further instructed to name those symptoms (-itis, -osis, -algia as in tendonosis) and then apply a therapy to those symptoms. This commonly is where their diagnosis stops.

Your health care provider follows a typical medical diagnostic flow chart. When something does not work, he logically tries something else guided by the flow chart. When that treatment fails to work, your doctor again tries something else, or does a more thorough diagnostic workup of the suspected problem region of the body using diagnostic tests.

Simply, this is why there are so many MRI scans of the knees, muscles and other regions when treatment fails and manual evaluation of the symptomatic part fails to yield helpful diagnostic information.

Unfortunately, this story often ends with a more aggressive approach that frequently includes higher-end surgical specialists whose recommendation, almost by definition, must be a surgical option.

The surgical fix is typically directed toward the symptomatic part of your body and may afford some relief... for a time. However, the true cause is often never looked for or evaluated if the symptoms are relieved. Often this creates a chronic condition that worsens and causes increasing problems as you age, damaging joints and affecting your quality of life. For proof of this, look at the growing business of knee and hip replacements, as well as other joints.

So why do we do it? We do it because the care is expected to relieve symptoms from both the health care provider's point of view as well as the view of the insurance company. If the symptoms are resolved, the belief is that the problem is also corrected, even though the cause had never really been addressed.

As many patients discover once they return to the activities that created the original pain, they experience symptoms not only in the original region that was the cause for the surgery, but also in areas that they did not know were related. Furthermore, as doctors explore each new symptom, which is again given a name and similarly treated in the hope of relief, the patient stands a pretty good chance of developing additional problems over time that can damage joints and create chronic pain syndromes because the cause of it all was neither understood, nor addressed.

This is the medical equivalent of sticking your finger in the wall in an attempt to plug a leak only to find another leak, and another, and another because the real problem- the root cause- is not the leak but the way the water pressure is distributed against the incorrectly built wall.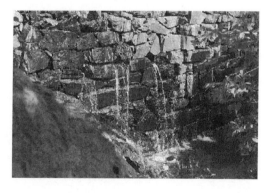

There is also another problem. Using this approach, as an area of the body malfunctions, you and I alter our pain sensitivity to accommodate to the functional deficit and the problem becomes chronic over time. This reduction of pain gives you, the patient a false sense of wellbeing since the true mechanical cause continues to exist without you being aware there even is a problem. After all, the cause may not be in the area of the pain at all. You will learn about this later in the book.

Meanwhile, since the pain medications used for mechanical problems provide relief from pain giving the patient a false sense of wellbeing, he cannot significantly improve function, even after traditional rehabilitation. As the patient ages, he is quite likely to experience increasing episodes of pain from related joints along the kinetic chains and are more likely to require joint replacements as their overly loaded joints become damaged beyond repair.

You have to wonder where the medical science is in all this madness.

Science is a system and means of acquiring knowledge using observation and experimentation to describe and explain phenomena. Science also refers to an organized body of knowledge gained using that system. Most health care providers believe their methods are scientific or at least based on science. This is not to be confused with usage of the scientific method that generally is accepted in all prominent health care professions.

Confused? I don't blame you. Think of it this way.

Many procedures done for the musculoskeletal system including back surgeries, shoulder surgeries and other body modifications have fallen out of favor. Only after enough procedures were performed and tracked over an extended period of time was it realized that these procedures caused more harm instead of helping the persons original problem.

This is largely because when a procedure becomes fashionable, many doctors learn to perform the procedure, believing they are alleviating suffering by treating the cause of the problem. This rapidly becomes the 'community standard of care' as more providers adopt the procedure so they are not violating 'community standards of care'.

Community standards are the way other health care providers practice in their geographic area. A deviation from the norm in a malpractice case can be used against the health care provider and is often the reason a malpractice suit succeeds. It is also why the majority of providers in a given geographic region practice similarly, even when a treatment can be found to be ineffective and possibly harmful.

An example of this was in the 1940's -1960s when it was believed the disc was the cause of back pain. Therefore, disc surgery was the 'community standard'. Countless people suffered from failed back surgery syndrome as a result while countless surgeons reaped the financial rewards[42].

Of course, in our current health care environment, these highly dangerous and invasive surgeries are no longer taken lightly and only performed when certain criteria are met for the best outcome. Today, there are many people helped by surgeries such as these; but if the true cause had been detected before the damage was done; it is less likely the patient would ever require this type of intervention at all.

As I stated before, science is a system and means of acquiring knowledge using observation and experimentation to describe and explain phenomena. Science also refers to an organized body of knowledge gained using that system.

Although health care practitioners are taught to look at lower back pain, neck pain and other types of joint pain in the body through scientific means, it does not mean their approach to diagnosis and treatment is based on strong science.

In other words, most studies on problems like back pain attempt to use the double blind method (http://en.wikipedia.org/wiki/Double-blind#Double-blind_trials) where neither the experimenters nor the assessors of the results, and not even the patients know which group is subject to which procedure. This is done to assure the results are free of biases and expectations that can influence the results.

Double blind testing methods works well historically for drug trials. When used on the musculoskeletal system, the results often leave us wanting information that is more conclusive.

This is because a patient's symptoms are subjective vs. objective. For instance, when a person fills out a pain questionnaire, if they have no pain and can function, these evaluation tools have them scoring low on the pain scale and high on the function scale.

This person may later have disabling pain due to a problem that was not noticed because the person accommodated their level of function or lack of function; and per their perception, had no discomfort or disability.

As this same person ages, the pain scale in the questionnaire stands a good chance of looking worse as their minimally symptomatic existing problems become more chronic and the joints and muscles become damaged over time.

An experienced musculoskeletal evaluator has a better opportunity than a non-trained musculoskeletal evaluator to pick up on malfunctions patients perceive as normal. For example, not being able to touch his toes, or having chronic knee pain when running causing her to use pain avoidance behaviors. Simply put, avoiding those activities that cause pain.

If you are someone with a body style issue, and most people are, over time you have acquired musculoskeletal adaptations that are only painful when the experienced health care practitioner properly evaluates you. Or, you may learn about these problems by accident when you lift up your child, reach for a dish from the kitchen cupboard, play sports or step wrong. At that time, you visit the doctor and say something like, "I was fine until I (whatever it was you did)."

Most health care medical personnel hear stories like this every day and if they are any good it, becomes an important part of the total history they gather during the initial consultation.

It is critical for health care practitioners to dig deeper for clues when evaluating problems in the musculoskeletal system because even though knee pain or shoulder pain may appear to come from the painful joint, as you are learning from this book, the cause is often in another part of the body. It is your health care provider's job to connect the dots.

Consultations should be intuitive and a doctor who truly understands the mechanisms behinds your symptoms will ask the right questions, even though they may not seem to relate to the pain itself. An 'enlightened practitioner' will look at the you, not be blinded by obvious symptoms, and make educated assumptions based on body style; trying all the while to figure out why the problem occurred in the first place. In other words, he is looking for the cause of the problem.

The 'enlightened practitioner' will ask pointed questions that go beyond the obvious and see if there is a correlation between body style issues and the symptoms you are experiencing. When your health care practitioner asks the right questions, you will describe a body roadmap that leads to a more appropriate diagnosis and treatment based on your observed body style.

A knowledgeable practitioner derives a tremendous amount of useful medical opinions from observing your body style alone. Added to the history you provide, he likely knows what the true cause is with a high level of certainty even before he performs a full evaluation on you.

How? Because it is quite rare for pain to just exist without a mechanical basis unless it is being referred via another mechanism such as chronic muscular or tendon dysfunction, inflammation such as Lyme Disease, Rheumatoid Arthritis, Gout or neurological involvement such as a disc herniation or tumor (which are possible but do not happen frequently), or organic disease such as cancer or infection. Most of these concerns are rare and only happen in a small part of our population.

In the case of tendon or chronic muscular involvement, there is almost always a mechanical cause. In the much rarer event of organic disease, typically the pain will not relate to body style and exacerbations often randomly appear, without provocation and may even wake you up in the middle of the night with unexplainable pain as well. While neurological pain often has exacerbations without provocation, disc herniation always has a mechanical cause. The cause must be evaluated and treated for optimal long-term results.

The majority of today's doctors are trained to make assumptions based on symptoms and disease processes rather than using a functional model. Based on this flawed training, most doctors assume that conditions are self-limiting, especially if the symptoms were reduced or eliminated without intervention, or with the use of prescription medication.

The patient who experiences pain relief may have accommodated the malfunction and appear to be free of pain because of increased tolerance that makes the pain less noticeable. This person risks going to the gym, loading up the malfunctioning area with weights or other exercise regimens and now has the pain return after the workout because the self-limiting pain was due to a body part (s) functioning poorly.

Usually the patient is told to ice or heat it, stay off it until it does not hurt anymore and then slowly return to activity. Often, the patient is told to constantly stretch the region for flexibility even though a properly functioning body part should not, under normal function, have the muscles surrounding the region tighten.

An example is the person who works out with the personal trainer.

The trainer has a lot at stake to help you achieve your personal fitness goals. Certain exercises, however, cause pain and soon the trainer is modifying the exercises to avoid the pain so you believe you are improving. Soon after, you find you cannot progress or develop a problem while working out and choose to stop working with the trainer.

The reality is the person has mechanical issues reinforced by the trainer accommodating to them. This is a type of pain avoidance behavior.

Building Healthy Musculoskeletal Relationships

The situation I just described doesn't help the client / soon-to-be-patient or the trainer. I regularly meet with many personal trainers (not to be confused with certified athletic trainers) and create relationships with Pilates instructors to educate them about the concept of leverage. Rather than modifying the training routine that enables the malfunction, they should consider partnering with a chiropractor or a highly skilled rehab therapist to rehabilitate the region so their client can now succeed in performing the exercises without modification.

Now, instead of a frustrated client unable to achieve her goal, setting the stage for future injury and a loss of business for the trainer, the outcome is very different. The client reaches her goals, gains strength and is often able to function at a much higher level mechanically than her body would have allowed before treatment.

As an added, but not unexpected bonus, she experiences fewer injuries and painful episodes in her back, neck and other body joints.

This is why it is critical that people understand the difference between pain relief and improved function. You will explore the difference in more detail later in the book when I discuss firing patterns and how your body mechanics works either for you, or against you.

Meanwhile, think about the last time you visited the local mall for an early morning walk during the oppressive heat of the summer or the arctic chill of winter; or just to go window shopping. Many people simply cannot tolerate that long walk in the mall because of back pain. The problem intensifies with age. Of course, when the pain seems lessened, everyone takes advantage and takes the walk.

When the pain returns, the walker assumes he reinjured the area or he overused it; when actually, the body area in pain was not the problem but merely a symptom of a greater mechanical issue elsewhere in the body.

Often as these problems become chronic the person avoids the aggravating activity (pain avoidance behavior) or sometimes wears appliances (knee braces, for instance) because it provides relief during the activity, although it does not truly help address the underlying cause of the pain. He typically stops scheduling appointments with his medical health practitioner, who naturally assumes his patient has improved.

The reality is that the patient gives up, avoids the activity or begins wearing an appliance that can make the aggravating activities tolerable. The truth is that over the years, the involved joints often become arthritic because of years of malfunction and the excessive wear. Sadly, the patient expects exactly this result and 'lives with it.'

Because of our current health care paradigm, as patients get older, they expect to degenerate, to rely on medications for pain and other health problems.

Based on our current way of practicing mainstream health care, why should we expect this to change?

Consider this; If we changed the paradigm to one that is more functional and less reliant on just symptoms; one that is more preventive and less reliant on medication and intervention, could we expect a different outcome as people get older? I think so. While there are chemical changes in the body as we age, improving the body mechanics of an aging public has the potential to markedly improve how we age and to improve our quality of life.

The Dysfunctional Musculoskeletal System Diagnostic Model

According to the American Board of Family Medicine, the primary care physician model we currently use has evolved in the United States since the 1960's.

"Once the new specialty of family medicine and its training programs were launched in 1969, innovative primary care leaders proposed classification systems to describe the work of family physicians and other primary care clinicians. Systematic descriptions of family medicine and primary care were established based on data developed and shared among practices." (http://www.jabfm.org/cgi/content/full/19/1/1)

These front line providers who are trained and schooled in emergency medicine and internal diseases are inadequately schooled in the proper diagnosis and treatment of the musculoskeletal system[43].

Many of the symptoms people present often overlap from the musculoskeletal to the organic disease realm, evaluated with blood tests, biopsies and procedures associated with today's mainstream medical practice.

A common example is stomach symptoms. Many people with stomach complaints visiting gastrointestinal specialists find out that both their upper and lower GI tests are negative. Many find themselves looking to internet sites such as www.wrongdiagnosis.com filled with these types of complaints.

In many cases, medications taken for the patient's other medical complaints cause the problem. Other times, the patient is 'diagnosed' with having irritable bowel syndrome or simply a muscle spasm.

These patients, who schedule appointments with me for back or neck complaints and, during the course of treatment have the abdominal muscle tightness addressed, frequently notice their GI symptoms resolve.

Does it sound like you are reading that one plus one equals a bushel of tomatoes?

Well, try this.

Many people with chronic lung problems also have musculoskeletal involvement due to labored breathing and joint malfunction in the rib cage affecting the expansion of the lungs. Correcting these functional issues can markedly improve a patient's response to care whereas the often-prescribed drug based 'solution' cannot improve the function of the ribs, pelvis and thoracic spine, which are commonly involved in breathing issues.

Unfortunately, primary care physicians rarely refer these patients to my office for a consult on these problems.

Fortunately, even without the referral, our office helps many patients suffering from the symptoms described. They come in for treatment of one complaint and experience marked improvements beyond what they experience in the offices of their pulmonary specialists.

Since, in our current health care system, musculoskeletal evaluation is often cursory or not considered at all, when a symptom profile appears to be disease orientated, most people are tested to rule out life threatening problems or referred to high-profile niche specialists.

> Doctors are ill equipped to offer a musculoskeletal diagnosis and treatment resulting in thousands of unnecessary MRI and diaganostic scans to try to find the cause of a patient's pain.

Few medical specialists (other than orthopedics or physiatrists because of their specialty) consider the involvement of the musculoskeletal system in their realm. Based on clinical experience, many of these medical tests such as upper and lower

GI could likely be avoided if medical providers considered the effect of the musculoskeletal system when ruling out disease processes, especially since most of their tests turn out negative and the musculoskeletal system is often the cause of the disease like symptoms.

Their focus on diseases without ruling out the musculoskeletal components often cause unnecessary secondary tests as well; and the concern for musculoskeletal involvement is typically secondary after the all the tests come back negative.

Manual evaluation and treatment of these areas from a functional perspective can help avoid many of the common tests currently performed because those who are experiencing symptoms due to musculoskeletal dysfunction will improve, often at a cost lower than the diagnostic test itself. This is great argument for treating and evaluating first, then running diagnostic tests only if the problem does not improve. This is also a great argument for the current systems to incorporate providers who treat and understand the musculoskeletal system while trying to evaluate as well as treat many suspected disease entities.

Many symptom complexes fall under what is termed "Somatic Disorders" and was studied and published in the Osteopathic literature[43]. Since many diseases are rare and occur infrequently, shouldn't health care providers know how to manually assess the musculoskeletal system first to rule out the medical necessity for many invasive and expensive tests? The AMA attempted to address this with resolution 310 in 2003[44]. Surveys and testing of medical students and residents suggest that opportunity and training in musculoskeletal medicine during medical school and residency are woefully inadequate.

This lack of adequate training in musculoskeletal diagnosis results in many patients placed on drugs for relief of their complaints their doctors failed to understand because they were ill equipped to understand..

The result: thousands of unneeded MRI and other advanced diagnostic scans to try to find the source of the pain[45]. The musculoskeletal system is tied to many symptom complexes of the internal organ systems. Health care providers who lack a great musculoskeletal skill set, or who have a personal bias that these types of symptoms must be organic are more likely to run tests with great costs to our health care system and little benefit to the patient[46].

Manual evaluation skills for the musculoskeletal system and a willingness to integrate with other health care disciplines that are not part of the 'traditional' medical model are essential if we are to reform properly our current expensive and symptom based health care system and offer patients real relief.

While ruling out life threatening conditions is a good thing, training that is more complete and better manual diagnostic skills would reduce the necessity for high tech testing. That just leaves the lawsuit fear factor.

The other reason for all the tests that might otherwise be unnecessary with a functional musculoskeletal evaluation are a litigious society. The overuse of tests occurs very much because from a liability standpoint doctors use these scans to rule out life threatening conditions in the absence of quality manual musculoskeletal evaluation skills.

If a doctor (especially an emergency room doctor) misses a life threatening condition, he would surely be a liability suit target. Doctors are safe when they follow community standards, even if the community standard is to run all these tests and not do a musculoskeletal workup.

A better manual skill set would be quite helpful in triage and may eliminate some diagnostic tests such as MRI scans. This would make patient evaluation more cost effective as well as diagnostically leading to recommending effective solutions in the emergency room.

Life threatening conditions occur in small portions of the population. A good manual evaluation of the musculoskeletal system in addition to the abdomen, heart and other vital systems should be part of your diagnostic workup before expensive tests are ordered.

The current system has trained patients to expect many tests to identify problems that are just not necessary. This additional skill would allow for much better diagnosis, direction with greater cost effectiveness during the ER visit.

I personally know a chiropractor who works in the emergency room of the Meadowlands Hospital in northern New Jersey. Initially, the physicians in the hospital did not know how a chiropractor could help some of the serious emergencies that can show up in the ER.

After some time, they now understand his value during assessment and treatment of those who came to the ER. Especially with patients complaining of severe back pain and chest pain, which are often confused with heart attacks, as well as the many other conditions that would otherwise have required expensive tests and diagnostics. Tests and diagnostics previously given that may have been avoided with a skilled musculoskeletal health care provider on site.

Since joining the hospital ER, my colleague estimates that he has saved both the hospital and its patients multiple thousands of dollars in tests while improving the quality of the ER experience for those in pain.

Years ago, when health care was simpler, the primary care doctors were skilled at manual evaluation with their hands. Much of this skill and knowledge has now taken a back seat to high tech tests due to the physician's reliance on today's diagnostic tools, which are a major driver of costs for health care[47].

Adding insult to injury, many of these tests yield meaningless information[48].

The use of flow charts for the musculoskeletal system in the absence of these skills is like looking for the light switch in an unfamiliar dark room. The use of medication to relieve conditions doctors do not understand require reevaluation because the initial symptom may have just been the beginning of a problem that, diagnosed correctly at the time, was curable.

Take osteoarthritis. Many people with gait related issues develop bad knees and degenerative spinal changes because the problem was that they hurt from time to time; and the underlying gait issue was never addressed. Ignoring the gait issue leads to permanent damage in their later years.

During the course of more than twenty years of practice, many patients had symptoms that have come and gone, decreased with medication that gives them a false sense of wellbeing. Years later, they learn of the damage done requiring either joint replacement or another surgical procedure.

For the majority of these patients, the surgical outcome could clearly have been preventable... if the original health care provider understood the initial symptoms and then been able to communicate to the patient experiencing the problem.

Treating Cause Vs. Managing Pain –

What's The Difference And Why Doctors Don't Think That Way

Have you ever wondered why the treatment of the back, neck, shoulders, knees, discs and related problems never has consistent outcomes? Why is it that certain people's joints last their entire lives yet other people have joints that simply go bad or wear out?

Historically, disc surgeries were performed on millions of people because of fashion trends in treatment rather than the science of why people have back problems.

It was at one time theorized by orthopedists that the lumbar disc was the cause of back pain, resulting in thousands of these surgeries being done based solely on a theory that became fashionable in the 1940's and 50's[49]. The result was chronic pain from failed back surgery because the true cause was never adequately understood or addressed. Life-long pain complicated by procedures that could have been avoided with a better understanding of the underlying mechanics leading to back pain.

Many painful conditions of the back, neck, shoulder, knees and hips have been treated using theories that were applied to the areas of symptoms, rather than addressing the functional causes due to a lack of understanding of why these conditions exist.

Many health care providers learn from the system to manage these musculoskeletal conditions as if they were degenerative diseases rather than mechanical problems. Since pain caused by movement is mechanical in nature, managing the pain rather than properly addressing the mechanism of the pain often leads to the problem worsening over time both in the way it feels and structurally. Longstanding mechanical problems are regularly interpreted in x-rays as arthritis and degenerative processes, rather than the mechanical problems these findings represent.

Abundant theories on pain and problem management have resulted in procedures that logically made sense on the surface. However, these theories did nothing to resolve the cause of the functional problems people experience during their lives because of the way they are built (body style). Instead, surgeries and procedures designed to relieve a symptom but failed in improving function are performed and, at its worst, leave people worse off than if they never had the problem treated[49].

Different groups of health care providers have attempted to treat problems of the neck, back shoulder and other joint related complaints. Each group applies its philosophy to the treatment methods based on the varying theories of how the problems occur.

These providers include physiatrists, rheumatologists, physical therapists, pain management professionals, occupational therapists, massage therapists and chiropractors.

Each group proclaims it has the best solution(s) for these problems. These solutions may include exercises, epidural injections, manipulation, Myofascial treatments including Graston technique, Myofascial release (Active Release Techniques ® being a style of this), traction, ultrasound, exercises, movement therapy, surgeries and more.

You have to ask, "Can every solution be correct?"

Is it possible for everyone to have different approaches and all get the desired outcomes without coming to similar conclusions on why the problem exists?

Some approaches just treat the painful region with medications, or attempt to exercise the painful part after applying different treatments to the region. Other approaches treat the mechanical problem that is behind it all.

As a consumer, you need to be able to tell the difference and choose carefully. Be warned, though, your doctor may or may not be a great help depending on his belief system which often will steer you toward other providers with a similar belief. Do you want to treat the cause of the problem, the symptom, or both? Moreover, can your health care provider tell the difference?

The pharmaceutical industry model is based on symptom relief and is reinforced by the medical community. Many medical doctors realize this and send their patients to chiropractors or therapists to help improve their patient's overall problem. However, many more medical doctors primarily rely on medications and refer people who do not get relief from the medications to orthopedic specialists who then refer the patients for whom they do not have a surgical option to physical therapists.

Are people being treated for pain with medication really better? Did we really understand why a part of their body became painful, or did we create a potential future problem by making a mechanical problem more chronic only to be dealt with more aggressively in the future?

Practical experience dictates that problems are only solved if you follow a logical path to its logical conclusion. If we conclude pain is the problem, then medications and testing different therapies on the painful part should work every time.

The reality is that treating painful symptoms has always yielded irregular results. We have hundreds of thousands of people who have experienced joint replacement and chronic pain in their joints as they age. In my experience, if you truly understand the basis of joint pain or the pain of a body part, your health care provider should be able to:

1. Explain the reason for the pain to the person rationally. *(I have often heard patients being told that they are in pain because they were older, they were arthritic, stuff happens, etc.)*

2. Demonstrate the dysfunction causing the pain to the patient. *(Most health care providers use static orthopedic tests for this, however, these tests often just confirm what you already know already; it hurts when you do that. Many of today's chiropractors and therapists are learning active evaluation methods that are much more effective in diagnosing and showing the dysfunction behind the pain.)*

3. Prescribe a treatment path that corrects the dysfunction and improves the way the body works. *(Rarely does that include an injection or a pill, but these modalities can help the process along by relieving pain allowing a better tolerance to treatment).*

The thought process behind a particular treatment is extremely important.

If you have shoulder pain and your health care provider just evaluates and treats the shoulder that hurts and recommends activity avoidance, it may temporarily relieve the pain. However, when you return to performing normal activity, the problem will return. Rest is rarely effective without first finding the true problem behind the pain.

> You can place a paintbrush in most people's hands but only a small fraction of them will produce art.
>
> It is the same with rehabilitation.

Beware, you've been trained to expect only the painful part to be evaluated and treated. With this approach, many end up with pain, more tests and surgery if tests show the chronic painful part is now been damaged over time.

You can place a paintbrush in most people's hands but only a small fraction of them will produce art. In the case of rehabilitation, you can teach thousands of doctors *how* to rehabilitate. However, unless you first teach them *why* problems occur and to look for the cause first, instead of trying to apply treatment to poorly understood symptoms, the treatment will often be inappropriate, expensive, risky, non-curative and lead to more chronic problems that can ultimately result in joint damage, surgeries and a less than desirable outcome over time.

Many studies attempt to quantify whether a particular treatment works for a particular ailment. By design, most studies of therapies used on painful conditions look at a specific treatment to the painful part to see if it relieves the pain based on certain strict parameters.

A great deal of these studies are incredibly restrictive, and due to study limitations usually do not reflect real-world treatments that can involve the use of different methods during treatment rather than just one particular treatment. The studies do, however, tend to focus on evaluating patient satisfaction rather than judging whether the thought processes used are right or wrong.

It is very common for lower back studies to operate this way, attempting to apply the double blind philosophy that many drugs use to physical medicine. The problem is that because of the nature of the musculoskeletal system, limiting the intervention to the painful part, or limiting the provider to a particular method often gives us inconclusive study results at best.

Another common example is studies that try to evaluate spinal manipulation against physical therapy. Often, although spinal manipulation is more effective in some studies and physical therapy is effective in others, most chiropractors use a combination of physical treatments, exercise and muscle work to get the desired results. Many physical therapists cross over as well, and may use manipulation in combination with their treatments. The lesson here is that limiting a profession's treatment in a study yields questionable data at best, since in the real world, practitioners take advantage of additional treatments to get their results.

Perhaps, we need to evaluate management philosophy as well as outcomes when the practitioner is told he cannot practice using all the tools available to him. Perhaps, we need to examine the role of management philosophy in determining the overall effectiveness of a treatment.

What is most interesting, though, is patient satisfaction. Chiropractors routinely have the highest level of patient satisfaction using their methods of treatment. This is important because satisfaction is generally an impression of the total therapeutic encounter; including the total patient experience.

Remember the April 2009, Consumer Reports? Patients stated that chiropractic care had the highest level of satisfaction compared to medical and physical therapy type providers[50] in a comprehensive study they performed. Could it be that a differently designed type of study for musculoskeletal complaints is more useful to the health care community than attempting double blind drug style protocols?

Moreover, what happens later? Are the patients treated in these studies asked how they are doing one, two or five years after the treatment or intervention? Are the interventions results still in place or was there only temporary relief? Many studies do not follow-up on the original population years later. Could it be we need a different paradigm for better evaluating interventions of the musculoskeletal system?

The Ethics Of Treatment

Isn't a functional method of evaluation and treatment more ethical, and how ethical is our current paradigm?

Paradigm and ethics are some of the largest cost drivers in the health care system. Ineffective treatment applied to poorly understood conditions is common. Since the current system teaches most health care providers about how to treat conditions instead of the mechanisms behind the problems, why should you expect better evaluations and treatment regimens for what truly ails you?

Is it ethical for medical doctors to treat what they do not understand? What is the criterion for an effective treatment? Understandably, most people want the symptoms of their problem resolved. They also want to be able to function in a way that minimizes the likelihood the problem will reoccur.

Understanding your problems can help you avoid surgical procedures that produce undesirable consequences for many people looking for relief of chronically painful conditions.

Our current system has taught the public to expect a symptoms management based approach; an approach I believe is the single most prevalent reason people experience chronic pain in their joints as they age. Is it any wonder many health providers in the medical field believe we should fall apart, degenerate, and suffer greatly as we age? I often wondered what it means to manage pain, manage a shoulder, manage back pain, or for that matter any other condition.

Managing pain *sounds* appropriate when someone is pain but is it appropriate to manage something as a health care provider if I do not understand why you are in pain? What exactly am I managing?

If any doctor gave you a pill, or an injection and the pain was gone until you went back to your activity, did that really work to resolve your problem or did you just get some temporary relief?

Is it appropriate if a doctor teaches you that it is okay to ignore your body; that pains are just pains without consequences; and that your parts are replaceable when they wear out? Is that really ethical?

Isn't it too late when years later, the joint is no longer viable , causing problems with the way you used to function and needs to be replaced or you will suffer with chronic pain and impaired mobility?

Could a more knowledgeable preventive approach when you were young prevented a lifetime of chronic pain and problems with your back and neck?

This is precisely why a functional approach is more appropriate when compared to the current symptom based approach.

With the symptom approach, you try the medication and see if it relieves the pain. If it does relieve the pain, you keep taking the medication because it must be working.

On what is it working? Is the pain the problem? Or is it really a consequence of body mechanics that few people in health care want to understand well enough to communicate to you in a way you can understand it?

Long-term usage of common medications such as Ibuprofen is not as safe as many people believe [51] and can damage the liver as well as other organ systems. Many of us have come to believe that over the counter medication is totally safe. However, it is really designed for intermittent use. The problems it creates costs more years down the road adding to our overall national health care tab. Prevention is less expensive and better for our quality of life.

Take a good look at all the medical care provider groups mentioned in this book who treat your painful condition and apply the currently acceptable and expected therapy- the community standard. Then look at the outcomes from these interventions. A patient can only conclude that unless you treat the underlying cause, he stands a very good chance of developing painful long-term problems.

Here's a different way of thinking about it:

Do our bodies degenerate, suffering joint pain and falling apart necessitating replacement parts *because* we get older?

Or, is it that the health care system, and your health care provider expects you to degenerate and fall apart as you age? That your medical practitioner wants you to experience increasing joint pain fulfilling his expectation, and expects you to become a candidate for joint replacement, fulfilling his purpose, all because the ignored joints become damaged during a lifetime of poor diagnosis and borderline neglectful treatment.

For thousands of health care providers, relieving the symptoms is treating the condition. Therein lays the problem with joint and chronic pain.

Don't get me wrong. There are situations where the pain is the actual problem. Then, and only then is it appropriate and perfectly ethical to treat the pain. Examples of this would be muscle pulls, surgical scars that are healing, sprains, auto immune and disease states affecting the joints of the body.

Dinosaur-Sounding Treatment

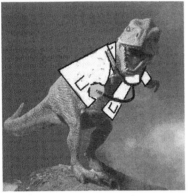

In the prehistoric world, the Allosaurus was an incredibly large and carnivorous dinosaur native to North America during the upper Jurassic period. Not unlike our description of the modern health care system and the community standard physicians who worship and feed it. Here's where this is going.

The predominant health care system in the western world (of which North America is a part) is allopathic medicine. Allopathic medicine treats disease symptoms with different remedies expected to produce different effects from those caused by the disease.

Most of today's health problems are treated with allopathic methods with varying degrees of success. For example, the allopathic symptoms based model may or may not work for diagnosing a gall bladder because symptoms of a damaged gall bladder are often unpredictable. There can be numerous attacks with symptoms that often imitate other conditions. Numerous tests, including ultrasound, may or may not yield a concrete diagnosis.

It is not unheard of for a surgeon to remove a healthy gall bladder because he thought the organ was diseased based on the symptoms. It has also been reported that some patients who had healthy gall bladders removed improved, leaving many who study the phenomenon to wonder if the relief was due to the sugar pill-placebo effect[52].

Symptoms may not relate at all to the problems you are trying to have evaluated and treated. However, poor function will consistently show itself using active evaluation methods and reproduce the symptoms.

This is especially true for problems in the musculoskeletal system.

Allopathic symptoms-based medicine has created all sorts of tests used to find causes for your problems. Focusing on the problem area because the area is painful, one of our modern and expensive high-tech Magnetic Resonance Imaging (MRI) or x-ray tests to the region often shows an identifiable problem. Evaluations with standard orthopedic tests are designed to provoke symptoms from the symptomatic region.

The problem is that these tests and evaluations do not look for why the body part or region has a problem in the region in question. This results in far too many unsuccessful treatment regimens and avoidable surgeries for painful shoulders, knees and other areas incorrectly thought to be the cause.

A good example of this is shoulder impingement surgeries done to remove pressure on the supraspinatus muscle which can be impinged by bone growth or posture.

Nobody questions why bone grew in the direction it did. No one questions why the patient's shoulder is leaning forward, creating the posture that made the problem possible.

The care is directed at simply surgically removing the impingement to remove the pain producing part. A different line of thinking may make surgery unnecessary. A different line of thought may resolve the issue without performing a surgical procedure. Following a non-surgical path of treatment the patient may eliminate other future body-mechanic related problems due to the same cause which went untreated with surgery.

In other words, the shoulder impingement is likely a result of compensation occurring in the body. The impingement is a response to how the body reacts to gravity and body structure with tightness in the muscles secondary to postural adaptation.

Many procedures like the shoulder impingement procedure were due to fashion instead of scientific efficacy. The procedures were accepted by the medical community and taught to other providers because people *seemed* to improve after the surgeries. However, widely accepted procedures are constantly discontinued because as post-surgical time passed, it is realized that the procedure has little or no long-term benefit. They suffer an allosaurically-speaking allopathic demise.

Another example is arthroscopic surgery for arthritic knees[52]. This commonly recommended and performed procedure was found to be ultimately worthless in helping people get relief of knee pain.

> Thousands of people have undergone the now known-to- be- worthless and expensive arthroscopic knee procedures for arthritic knees.

According to the July 2002 issue of the New England Journal of Medicine, more than 650,000 people seeking relief from knee pain undergo arthroscopic procedures each year at an average cost of $5,000 per procedure. The study questioned the physiological proof that arthroscopy cures osteoarthritis and found none. In fact, people underwent these now known to be worthless and expensive procedures, its affiliated costs and eventual disability necessitating a recommendation for joint replacement just a few years after the procedure.

A different approach may have saved those knees from these consequences had it been considered during the years the person believed Advil® or a similar pain reliever was the answer to their problems.

Instead, a typical medical workup for back or neck pain in our current health care system includes a history related to the pain, evaluating the painful part and seeing how you function with the part in question. Ouch.

Your health care provider should at least have some very basic knowledge of the joint from anatomy classes and from his internship. He should understand what normal looks and acts like, and be able to either send you for an MRI or give you a referral to an orthopedic group. Alternatively, he should be prepared to do both if he does not understand the cause of your pain… the reason your pain exists.

The reality is that it is more common for your primary care physician to give you a prescription for pain medication during the visit than a referral to an orthopedist, chiropractor or other rehabilitation specialist. It is a close second to be sent for an MRI.

Then, your doctor delivers the bad news (how often do you get a call back with good news?) or gives that distinct privilege to visit the orthopedist (if you're referred). This is nothing new to you. Here's what you may not realize...

Many of the MRIs ordered never reveal the actual cause of the problem. The MRIs only confirm the damage that currently exists and show a history of poor function.

Therein is the problem. Very few orthopedists with whom I have ever met look past the symptomatic painful part. They merely screen people for pathology or problems to which they can recommend a surgical solution. Occasionally, they offer an injection to the problem area to relieve the pain. Unfortunately, patient results vary widely and may or may not actually receive any relief from the pain.

Instead, what usually happens is that upon review of the MRI results, the orthopedic surgeon wants to stay involved if he sees a surgical option is available. If not, he typically sends you, as fast as he can, to a physical therapist with instructions to rehabilitate the painful area and only the painful area. When the patient does not improve, he is likely given the "choice" of a more aggressive surgical option, if the MRI supports it.

One patient recently told me that she had three separate visits for problems all on the same side: one for her knee, one for her ankle and another for her hip.

This is outrageous and there is a better way! These are interconnected joints! Part of the kinetic chains! The knee, ankle and hip need evaluation as a group to understand the painful condition and the mechanism behind it. The rehabilitation of the area must address the entire problem, rather than just the knee pain which if commonly done.

To my chiropractic line of thinking, you first work to eliminate the pain *and* the mechanical causes of the problem with active evaluation, manipulation, joint and myofascial rehabilitation. Only if you fail to improve with rehabilitation do you return to your doctor for alternative recommendations, which can include prescription medication or a more aggressive surgical option.

Although there are small groups throughout the country that have begun to embrace the profession and its benefits, most orthopedic doctors do not refer patients to chiropractors. Maybe they fear non-surgical solution competition. However, a few recognize that chiropractors can help many difficult-to-manage patients who are not surgical candidates improve markedly when other methods, including physical therapy, fail. Today, there are even cases where chiropractors and orthopedic doctors work in the same offices, helping patients achieve their goals, in most cases non surgically.

Teaching Physicians to be "Doctors of Cause"

Health care providers learn that the more effective the evaluation is, the more likely it will lead to a more effective treatment. That is the problem. That also is why we must get away from the symptoms based disease model for the muscular and skeletal system. We must move toward teaching a functional based mechanical model that does not exclude disease processes, but is not obsessed with them.

While definitely not a physician, in her controversial book "Ageless," Suzanne Somers did write something of real importance; to find a "Doctor of Cause." Not a "Doctor of Symptoms." Finding a "doctor of cause" is more than a well-coined phrase.

This means you need to find doctors who know how to look outside the allopathic symptom box. You might have a hard time, though. In my experience, a doctor capable of thinking that way is a rarity. But, when dealing with problems of the human frame (back, legs, knees, hips, neck, shoulders, mid back), looking outside the community standard allopathic box helps solve everyday problems that symptoms doctors often cannot resolve effectively or cost effectively.

If solving your pain problem is not enough incentive, focus again, for a moment, on the financial problem.

The current symptom-disease model has been a very expensive way to treat an aging population. Increasing health insurance costs are constantly being blamed on our aging population. We need to stop falsely believing that each part of the body is its own separate department. Repeatedly we see that the human body is the sum of its parts and must be diagnosed and treated with this in mind. The idea in American health care that a physician can super-specialize in a specific niche area needs serious rethinking. It is time to stop looking at the symptom, to stop looking only at the part and ignoring the big picture.

Princeton economist Uwe Reinhardt believed that these rising expenses are all due to high tech 'solutions' and salaries that continue to balloon. She estimates that over the age of 75, we spend five times more on health care than when we are 40 years old. She also notes that compared to Japan, who spends much less per person at 75 years of age, U.S. patients are much more expensive without receiving a benefit[53].

Of course, you must consider a good deal of this cost is prescription drug related or fraud driven. However, could it be the Japanese paradigm for health care makes more sense? That, perhaps, less is more?

While I am not suggesting that older people should be deprived of needed care, I am concerned that our cradle-to-grave concept of health care needs to be rethought[54].

Is A Better Primary Care Physician Possible?

If you are old enough, you may remember the old small town doctor. If not, go rent the Kevin Costner film, "The Field of Dreams" for a look at the small town doctor played by Burt Lancaster. You do not get a medical education, but you do understand that this doctor knew his patients very well.

Years ago, better-trained generalists with manual evaluation skills second to none were reliable diagnosticians that got it right more often than not based entirely on experience and the ability to evaluate with just their hands, stethoscope's and minds. As you might have guessed, costs in those years for health care were markedly lower.

Contrast this with today's primary care providers who have a different skill set, minimal assessment tools, order multiple tests and refer you to other specialists who just look at only the part you are complaining about instead of all of you. For your trouble, you might learn the name of what your physician thinks best describes your condition and, if you are really lucky, a promise of an effective course of treatment with yet another referral.

The Health Care Crap Shoot

If health care providers are supposed to be so good at what they do in health care, why are patient results so uneven? Why is it that three doctors cannot agree on why you are in pain? Why do you need back or neck surgery and why did those body parts go bad? More importantly, was the pain and surgery preventable.

What happens when you ask the health care provider why you are in pain?

- Do you hear, "The MRI was positive."
- Do you get a blank stare and shoulder shrug.
- Does your doctor actually say, "I don't know."
- Are you told, "You're getting older. That stuff happens."

> If you have ever heard answers like these, it is time to shop around for a new doctor...
>
> He does not understand why you are in pain.
>
> In addition, a doctor can't treat something he doesn't understand and cannot quantify.

How about this insanity... Has anyone of your health care practitioners considered placing you on anti-depressants after they have failed to relieve your pain?

Not very good answers are they. The one thing all doctors universally understand is that you are in pain and you want a result that gets you out of pain, fast. This is why a traditional first method of treatment from most doctors in the medical system includes pain medication. Pain relief, however temporary, is a concept all health care providers understand well!

If you are hearing (or ever heard) answers like these, it is time to go doctor shopping again because they do not understand why you are in pain and a doctor cannot treat something he does not understand and cannot quantify.

Doctors are taught in school, to look at the condition in front of them, not necessarily the person with the condition. In some circles, this is changing. There are a few internship programs where students are labeled with a condition, placed in a room as a patient and undergo the tests that a real patient would need to experience. This is a quick way to teach developing health care providers to have empathy for those they evaluate and treat.

Our Diseased Disease-Based Health Care Paradigm

Our current United States health care paradigm tends to be disease based; and it is quite likely your doctor sees things through blinders, the limited and focused sight of his specialty. For example:

Your internist sees every muscular problem as a disease to treat with pain and anti-inflammatory medications and send you for an MRI of the region if the pain does not yield sufficient improvement to rule out a spinal degenerative disease.

The rheumatologist sees everyone with chronic pain as having a systemic disease. He automatically wants to rule out diseases such as rheumatoid arthritis, Fibromyalgia, or other diseases our body may have that creates inflammation and pain.

A cardiologist sees every episode of chest pain as a cardiac event even though many episodes can be attributed to rib based pain or muscle spasm due to a malfunction on other areas of the spine.

A gastrointestinal specialist sees every stomach complaint as an organic disorder and tests everyone with upper and lower GI tests, even though most of these are negative and can often have a musculoskeletal origin.

Each of these specialists have little or no training in the musculoskeletal system[55]. Instead, their patient goes through numerous, sometimes-intrusive tests. The patient is prescribed a frightening variety of sometimes-conflicting medications. Finally, if the patient shows no sign of improvement after trying these approaches, he is often told to just live with it or as I have seen, been given a frightfully expensive drug only affordable as long as the insurance company pays for it.

Depending on his philosophical background and thought process, a chiropractor sees a muscular problem as a spinal or body alignment issue. A sports chiropractor or other specialty chiropractor may see this as a gait issue or other type of problem. Unless something more serious is presented, each will try manipulation and gauge results over the course of a few visits before ever considering subjecting you to expensive and intrusive tests and medication 'therapy.' Many people improve and experience less pain after this type of intervention.

The Patient as Part of the Problem

I am going to share something here that you may have difficulty understanding or believing.

You, the patient, may not be very helpful to the doctor; and in not being helpful, you give him carte blanche to proceed with whatever tests and medications he likes even when it doesn't make sense.

You see, if you have had a body style problem for years, you consider certain aches and discomforts normal, even when it is not based on your previous experiences.

For example; if you have always been inflexible, you consider this normal because your uncle, your dad and your sister and other people in the family tree also are inflexible. Uncle Tom may have had back surgery, Aunt Nettie may have had had a bad hip, Uncle John had both knees replaced. Since people like this surround you and it is the norm for the people to whom you are related, you consider this normal.

> As a patient, you are part of the problem. You may not be very helpful to the doctor; and in not being helpful, you give him carte blanche to proceed with whatever tests and medications he likes.

Then, one day you bend over to pick something up off the floor and experience acute and excruciating back pain. It is no longer the 'normal' stiffness with which you are familiar.

Actually, that normal stiffness isn't normal at all.

As you read this book, you may start developing the opinion that there is a reason our spines, knees and other joints wear out and need replacement; that the reason is neglect rather than normal and expected. That's good. However, there is more…

It is quite plausible that many of the things from which we suffer and take for granted actually happens because of the way you are built.

To appreciate fully this new concept, you must understand that our body style and build determines how we function in life.

A doctor less knowledgeable or a friend who has maybe experienced lower or upper back problems himself may tell you that stuff just happens; to give it a few days and it will go away; it will "work itself out".

Many of my patients come from the "maybe it will go away" school of suffering and show up with chronic problems when they get older... and it no longer goes away.

What does go away mean, anyway? Does the problem go away? Do the over the counter for temporary relief medications no longer give temporary relief? Could this have been prevented if you were properly screened as a child in school for problems in body style and the way we walk, stand and move?

I have trained certified athletic trainers to look at their student athletes' body style issues. Those I have worked with agree that along with the annual scoliosis screening, the extra minute in evaluating body style and feet can very likely help millions of children avoid or significantly reduce problems, pain and suffering in the back, neck, shoulders and spine as they age.

> Your body style and build determines how you function.

Increasing the Odds of Finding Effective Care for Your Pain

Spinal and extremity manipulation (most commonly used by chiropractors and some Osteopaths in the North America) is a natural for dealing with body style issues. The manipulation of the joints helps restore both symmetry and normal movement, and directly addresses the spinal and extremity joint mechanics directly through the adjustment or manipulation.

Many health care practitioners who regularly use manipulation now also perform myofascial treatment to loosen tight areas and improve the function of the myofascial components surrounding joints.

Myofascia:

Fibrous tissue that encloses and separates layers of muscles; sheath of connective tissue.

They then use exercises to strengthen these formerly tightened regions so they are less likely to tighten again, while improving muscular coordination that decreases the likelihood of retightening.

This approach is most effective for the practitioner who looks at the entire body, not just the areas of main complaint, since the cause of pain in many cases may not originate in the area of complaint.

Health care practitioners who learn to look at body style, its effects and look outside the "symptom box" can more accurately diagnose why a problem occurred and offer a more effective long-term solution for the musculoskeletal system.

Trigger Points:

A stimulus that sets off an action, process, or series of events; an automatic or manual pulse or signal for an operation to start.

Some of the brightest people in the back pain business who understand how this works are able to look at a person, and with a high degree of accuracy, based entirely on body style, tell the patient what he suffers from before the patient even says anything.

This is possible because body style issues have predictable effects on function. Therefore, you can predict tendencies toward painful conditions with a high level of accuracy. Practitioners who truly understand function and dysfunction have a huge advantage for the patient in accurately treating and, in many cases, resolving long-term painful conditions others cannot resolve.

Dr. Janet Travell (http://en.wikipedia.org/wiki/Janet_G._Travell), a well-regarded and published researcher in myofascial treatment for Trigger Points was able to do this very accurately by those who had the privilege to hear her speak in the 1990's.

She was able to look at people and tell them what their problems likely were based on how they sat or stood; and she was often right in her assertions.

Fascinated with the concept of the predictability of prevention and treatment based on the role body mechanics has in our daily functions; I worked diligently to develop and document this same skill.

Based on seminars I've given, I believe all health care practitioners can be taught how to do this. The net effect is that health care provider inter reliability improved markedly because the doctors I taught now described

> **All health care practitioners can learn how to do this.**

mechanical dysfunctional patterns, rather than symptom specific conditions we are currently taught to describe. Health care providers would diagnose patient issues more accurately resulting in better and more cost effective treatment. Gone will be the days of differing diagnosis for shoulder pain from different health care providers for the same condition.

Here's how it helps. Body styles have known and predictable consequences in the human frame with which today's physicians are unfamiliar. They are, however, familiar with symptom-disease diagnosis and treatment.

The symptom and problem orientated approach we use today is very consistent in creating very irregular outcomes, frustrating the public and creating unneeded suffering.

The knowledge is available to change. However, as long as the current health care system teaches doctors the disease process and that each condition of the human frame is discrete (except when there is a well-documented injury) there will be no change. We must, instead teach the concepts of body style and mechanics and how to link it all together. Otherwise, treatment of the ailments that affect the human frame will be continue to be a costly hit or miss proposition in both human and financial terms.

Those of you who have been through typical back pain treatment understand. You go to your health care provider and may receive different prescriptions for medication; varying opinions regarding the use of heat, ice, and rest; muscle stimulation; injection; physical rehabilitation with exercises; chiropractic adjustments; spinal decompression tables; surgeries; etcetera, etcetera, etcetera.

Your doctor isn't the only source of confused treatment. You probably have a preconceived notion of what you should do for the condition based on what you heard on the radio; about a method you saw on the evening news that works; or from a legitimate story or advertorial you read in the newspaper. Maybe you think you know something based on a health care provider's recommendation, a referral from a friend, or a previous experience.

True, some of these methods are shown more effective than others in studies, but in your mind, as a patient, the recommended back treatment worked or it didn't.

Most primary care doctors, including pediatricians, understand little about the lower back and why it goes bad. However, they do have their theories based on their professional bias.

Many are taught by drug representatives and in seminars to use rest, heat and medications. After a short period of time, if the symptom has not gone away, many often think of sending a patient to an orthopedic surgeon who will run tests and may send you for therapy. And, although this continues to be the exception, some occasionally send you to a chiropractor.

Unfortunately, except in the case of being referred directly to a chiropractor, this diabolical medical dance has the effect of many people having unnecessary and expensive procedures, including back surgeries, with little benefit.

I regularly see a number of medical doctors as patients who themselves are victims of this thought process having had surgeries that placed them on disability instead of back in their offices.

An obstetrician who injured her neck in an auto accident, eventually had multiple surgeries recommended that left her with limited function and out of practice. She was a mess when she finally found her way to my office. With multiple surgeries and many (shudder) permanent changes, I did what I could to help. However with the multiple permanent changes made, it is difficult to reverse a poor course of care decision like this.

I was able to help her to the point any chiropractor would be able under the conditions; and then she returned to what she knew and what she was emotionally comfortable with- more specialists and procedures. Why? Because in her mind, the answer to her problems had to be found using 'serious doctors' who use 'serious' and often risk-laden procedures. Those same procedures that created her current, barely manageable condition.

Many procedures and diagnosis regimens to diagnose the disease process are laid out on flow charts, including problems in the back, neck, shoulders and other regions related to the back and extremities. The flow charts typically pertain to a condition a health care provider is attempting to diagnose and designed as a guide to help the practitioner diagnose a condition.

Having a flow chart to follow is not a bad idea. It can be helpful and my profession uses them as well. A reminder. A consistent way to move through a diagnosis process.

Unfortunately, most practitioners do not look outside these charts because they were never taught that you could, or that you should. I have treated many more doctors than just the obstetrician who is a victim of this philosophy.

In my opinion, the musculoskeletal system can use flow charts, but the flow charts need modification, and health care practitioners need educating to look beyond the obvious.

Take, for example the typical assessment and treatment of back pain. In the treatment of back pain, your health care provider assumes a diagnosis and a trial of treatment. The flow chart for chiropractic lower back treatment in my profession may say two-to-three weeks at three visits per week and reevaluate at that time. If the response is good (50 percent improvement), then "do this". If the response is poor or the person exacerbates, "do this" (usually MRI).

The flow chart says nothing about checking other regions of the body; gait or firing patterns, but expects us to use a diagnostic procedure if our result of care is poor. Usually, a poor result is because of a serious underlying cause such as an issue with a disc aggravating the problem.

We then perform our MRI if the patient does not improve and use this to justify a referral, change the treatment method or as verification of our assumptions if the patient begins to finally respond to care.

Following the flow chart as it is, doctors hope to guide a patient down the proper path of resolution, but what if all the tests are negative and the problem we are treating is due to another issue not seen by the chart? As you can see, there needs to be a way to look outside the box that is not currently on the treatment flow chart diagnostically. We need a more open train of thought with the musculoskeletal system to help people better.

Do you remember our earlier discussion about the inconsistency among physicians regarding patient assessment and treatment of the musculoskeletal system? Well, treatment of back pain that is really a symptom of another condition altogether is a common cause of irregular and unpredictable outcomes for patients.

Back pain is almost always related to a gait issue arising from how you are built and the way you walk. We see uneven results because the flow chart does not tell a doctor to look at gait and body style when treating back pain. Our schools teach doctors to treat the back, the disc, the joints, the sciatic pain as if the pain is the problem and the condition, rather than being a symptom of the way we move and walk. So, what is your doctor treating and what type of result can you reliably expect from such treatment when the symptomatic part rather than the true cause of the pain is treated?

About half of the visits to primary doctors are for painful conditions of the musculoskeletal system. Having musculoskeletal complaints handled with a disease mentality has undesirable side effects including drug reactions, expensive procedures that may not be helpful or may only address the symptom while leaving the cause unattended, never ending therapy, and patients whose conditions will predictably deteriorate as they age.

If you ask many people about their golden years, you hear about their bad knees, hips, and other joints that developed over time due to age.

If we had a way of thinking better, could we be aging be better? Could joints last a lot longer and perhaps last as long as we do? Do they have to go bad? What isn't our pediatrician telling us as we grow up? Are our growing pains really growing pains or are they really a sign of biomechanical problems that are being ignored because my primary doctor does not have the tools to understand what I am feeling or why? What is truly preventive care and what can I do for my children so they do not experience similar problems?

The answer is that if your health care provider does not functionally understand what he is treating, gives it a big medical sounding name and cannot give you some understanding of how the problem occurred that makes sense, he cannot possibly treat it reliably. He is simply throwing therapies at a problem hoping that something sticks using heat, ice, rest, ultrasound, medication, injections or exercise and in the worst cases, recommending surgery. Using this approach, we are doing the wrong thing for the person who needs our help.

When I treat a patient and they tell me what they are feeling, I can show them why they are feeling it. Unless there is something underlying the symptoms other than mechanical dysfunction such as a disc problem irritating a nerve, cancer, organ dysfunction, joint damage, disease processes that are all quite rare when compared to pain from gait issues; just about all the patients improve markedly.

The real test, of course, is the test of time. Does the work allow the patient to feel and function better for one month, two months, forever?

How often does the dental and periodontal patient return for interventional care for chronic tooth or gum issues? Body structural issue is similar to someone needing periodical dental care.

Emotional Stress and its effects on Myofascial Function and Pain

In 2002, Dr. John E. Sarno created a stir of interest introducing theories on the role that emotion plays in the back pain equation in his book "Healing Back Pain."

His colleagues in the department of rehabilitation had treated numerous people with varying levels of success. As referenced in his book, when he dealt with the emotional component of lower back and musculoskeletal pain, people were able to experience a resolution of chronic back pain and tightness that has lasted for years.

Dr. Sarno referred to the stress-related condition known as Tension Myofascial Syndrome (TMS). His theory does not take into account a mechanical disposition to pain but instead relies on convincing the reader how psychological therapy benefits those who suffer with chronic pain noticing a documented hormonal response to stress that causes muscles to tighten, as well aggravating a preexisting condition.

While it is likely that his treatment works on this component, it completely ignores a person's structural predisposition to pain. Further, his book does not detail the actual therapeutic methods employed by either his department or his office, but does try to lead the reader to believe that emotion plays a part in chronic pain. In part, and only in part, I agree with him.

In truth, stress does increase the tension of muscles and creates pain when the muscles become tighter due to the body's natural hormonal and neurological response to stress. Many of our patients do experience this and it is quite likely you have as well. Our reactionary sympathetic nervous system assures this through what is known as the "flight or fight response." This system prepares the body for action in response to stimulus whether it is to flee a predator, pounce on prey, or wake to greet the waiting morning.

Unfortunately, Dr. Sarno's book deals entirely with emotional stress. Missing is a thorough discussion of the body mechanics that created the problems his patients were having. Gait asymmetry predisposes the human frame to inappropriately increased forces on its structures. The greater the asymmetry of the body, the greater the *mechanical* stress which can lead to pain and breakdown in the ankles, knees, back, shoulder, neck and arms over time. When foot flare and asymmetry is more pronounced, the stress that affects these structures is greater.

Stress aggravates these underlying problems because it increases the strain on the joints as the muscles on the existing problematic structure become tighter. Chronic pain problems therefore become worse because of the autonomic nervous system, also known as the sympathetic nervous system, and its action on the muscles. Increased tension strains the spinal, pelvic, extremity and rib joints further creating chronic pain and negatively affecting movement. Emotional stressors often include work, traffic, job loss, arguments with children or spouses as well as too many other reasons to list here.

The other type of stress Dr. Sarno did not include is mechanical stress from exercise or just daily activities. The real question of course is that if stress causes chronic back pain, why isn't everyone who is experiencing a high amount of stress experiencing chronic back pain?

What differentiates those who are in chronic pain and respond to his therapy, those who do not respond and those who have no complaints but have a huge amount of emotional stress?

If stress does create chronic pain, practically everyone would be in pain during the most stressful times in his or her lives. After all, many people under stress experience greater tension and tightness in their muscles but do not find themselves with chronic back pain.

This topic has a place in this book because stress will aggravate an existing mechanical condition, usually through the body's use of hormones and neurological developmental mechanisms that have evolved over the years to improve the survivability of the species. However, stress is not the cause of chronic pain; it merely causes the muscles to tense because of a hormonal and neurological adaptive response, which tightens an already straining and dysfunctional musculoskeletal structure. Cause and effect must be kept in perspective. Musculoskeletal pain and its related dysfunction is generally an effect, and the body's foundation (our body style and the way we stand) is often the cause.

Recently, I went to the New Orleans Jazz festival with a group of friends my bother organized. During our first dinner conversation, I mentioned I was writing this book and talked about its point of view on pain.

One of the women at our table had visited Dr. Sarno after reading his book. She told me that a session with the doctor was $1000 dollars and that his patients could visit groups he established on an unlimited basis to "retune" if they forgot how to self manage using his psychologically based method.

I remember that she felt good in certain positions and felt uncomfortable while sitting or in other positions. When standing for too long she felt back pain and needed to sit down. I also recall noticing that she had obvious poor foot posture, gait asymmetry and when she stood there was an obvious distortion in her hips. As I typically do, I did point this out to her and she confessed that many of the shots, meds, rehabilitation regimens and other methods she used did not work for her to alleviate the condition until she visited Dr. Sarno. Apparently, none of her health care previous health care providers noticed her visually apparent mechanical issues or addressed them correctly for her to find a successful treatment regimen.

This story only further solidifies my opinion on Dr. Sarno's work, and work like his that ignores the mechanical and focuses on the psychological. While this is a form of pain control that is effective for some people, it is likely this patient will have knee, foot and upper back problems in the future because nobody really understood the underlying cause of her having chronic back pain, including Dr. Sarno and his work does not address this either.

We are all consumers in our health care system, it is vitally important that we understand our bodies better. Pain brings out emotions of fear, shortness of temper, irrational actions and frustration. I have treated many patients who underwent expensive tests, inappropriate therapies and surgeries; many of which are not reversible because of fear, desperation and irrational thinking regarding their condition. A panicky patient often places pressure on his physician to perform tests or procedures even if they are against the health care provider's better judgment. Health care providers attempt to satisfy their patient's needs to the best of their ability to understand. Whether or not you need it, most will refer you for tests if you ask them to.

That is not always the right thing to do. Instead, find doctors who think holistically and functionally (looking at everything and not just the symptoms), and you will be rewarded with a better health care experience including more cost effective care, fewer tests, fewer drug reactions and a better quality of life.

What Is The Right Type Of Care And The Right Type Of Health Care Provider For The Musculoskeletal System?

Unbelievably, there are doctors of many disciplines who taught themselves to look outside the box in their specialty. A more worldly approach looks at all possibilities, not just the obvious ones. Some attend seminars to learn how to think this way and others like me question what they have already learned and challenge it on a daily basis.

Health care professionals should regularly question what they do, why they do it, how they can do it better and look for ways to get outcomes that are more consistent.

Many of the sports doctors with whom I associate have learned various ways to evaluate outside the box and regularly attend seminars to improve their knowledge and find out what works best in resolving some of the most complex conditions.

In order to excel in the evaluation and treatment of the musculoskeletal system, you need to use active evaluation techniques that challenge areas of the body with force through painful or dysfunctional movement.

Active evaluation methods, a developing trend is beginning to replace many of the passive methods we learned in school, called traditional orthopedic tests (although some of these test are still valuable tools in evaluating problems). The health care provider observes what happens to the area when stressed by movement or certain motions, and acts upon those areas to improve functionality. A poorly functioning region recruits in other muscles, or not be able to develop enough force to resist causing pain, which indicates a dysfunctional region. The provider then treats the area based on his impression of the problem and then retests the region to see if it reacts differently, or if the pain has decreased significantly. This method yields information that is far more useful more consistently, leading to a better and more reliable outcome at the end of the visit.

Here is an example of an effective active test I use to evaluate shoulder function. While seated, the patient pushes with his palms open against my hands the following five ways: forward, upward, lateral, downward and across his chest.

This test evaluates mechanical advantage, muscular coordination and recruitment. To illustrate recruitment; I ask someone to push their hand against mine and their shoulder blade tightens into the neck on that side. In this example, a poorly functioning shoulder has brought in surrounding muscles, which substitute for poor mechanical advantage of the joint. The effect of a dysfunction such as this would be tight shoulders, neck and shoulder pain and even headaches because of the muscles used improperly. A positive active evaluative test, something both the patient and the health care provider can see, is weakness, shaking and lack of strength or force in the direction the person pushes.

A patient under standard static orthopedic protocols would endure certain tests while the health care provider provokes the joint for pain. These types of tests are what most health care providers learn in school in order to take their boards. However, unlike the active test that tells us if a joint is functioning well or poorly and then gives us an idea where to look next, the orthopedic test usually just confirms that something hurts or feels awkward. It also may be a reliable clue that the joint is damaged (tears of the glenoid labrum in the shoulder).

Orthopedic tests often lead to imaging tests that can lead to surgeries. On the other hand, the other tests I perform are the gateway for other non-invasive evaluations. The active tests I perform typically lead to mechanisms of injury and malfunction. The orthopedic tests often lead us to areas that are painful, and unless we have a history that is quite specific to an injury, does not help us determine how the injury occurred; or if there were problems prior to the damaging forces being applied to the now damaged joint.

Using the active evaluation technique I practice, many patients' chronic functional problems are more accurately diagnosed and most likely resolved at a lower cost with fewer office visits.

An enlightened health care practitioner who looks outside the box looks not just at your problem area. He looks at all of you.

- How you stand.
- How you walk.
- How you hold your upper body while sitting and standing.
- He evaluates your foot posture.

An enlightened practitioner takes a thorough history and almost instinctively knows what to ask based on typical symptom patterns that occur due to body style issues which are visually observed.

With knee pain, for example, he will ask about your feet, shins, back, neck and other areas that can be affected. He will ask you questions that may not seem relevant to your main complaint. However, based on your initial history intake form they know what they are looking for.

While someone with a body style issue may be totally unaware of any problem in other parts of their body, it is the health care practitioner's job to consider even problems that seem insignificant to the person who has the complaint. This can include occasional leg cramps, chronic neck tightness that is not painful, inflexibility, and the occasional back or knee pain that the patient does not think is a problem but may actually be.

In my experience, most people do not consider many complaints that seemingly come and go to be of any consequence. Most people believe the pain is the problem until you explain why it is often just the tip of the iceberg.

An out of the box evaluation is a combination of observation, history, asking the right questions, evaluating the patients intake sheet diagrams and watching them walk and move. A person's body style makes them more likely to experience problems such as back pain, neck pain and other musculoskeletal complaints. You can only assess the body style by looking at the patient as a whole.

A thorough practitioner matches up your history and evaluates your body style to see if his assumptions based on your body style match up with your historical complaints. If they do, the mechanical cause of your pain can be confirmed during the evaluation, with the practitioner being able to create certain assumptions on what they would likely find.

An active evaluation uses provocative tests, feels muscular spasms, restrictions of movement, checks ranges of motion, and tests the way muscle groups interact when forces are placed upon them. The collective process allows a health care practitioner to see why your complaint exists, and places real life forces into the region to assess what happens with those forces placed upon the body.

By simulating what you do daily with your regular lifestyle, exaggerated by resistance, a knowledgeable health care practitioner can visualize movement dysfunction, recruitment of inappropriate muscles and diagnose a mechanical process that causes chronic pain much more effectively when compared to standard orthopedic tests. Providers who evaluate this way may still use some of the standard orthopedic tests; however, they are likely to be used only occasionally.

An example of a useful standard orthopedic test is Lachman's. Lachman's is used to evaluate a knee injury and figure out if the patient damaged the cruciate ligaments in the knee. This is a situation where static tests are better since we often more clearly see an unstable joint.

If an area is functioning poorly, it likely has muscular and sometimes ligamentous tightness surrounding the areas being evaluated. Your doctor would also see complimentary tightness in other areas that respond in kind.

For example, in the lower back, with foot flare, typically we see a tightening of the oblique muscles in the abdominal region when tested. Secondarily, we see a tightening of the quadratus lumborum on the opposite side, multifidii on the same side, psoas on the opposite side, quadriceps on the opposite side, hamstring and gastroc on the same side.

> **Lachman's Test:**
>
> The examiner has the patient lay on his back with his knee bent at 30 degrees.
>
> Holding the end portion of the patient's thigh with one hand and the top of the shin with the other hand, the examiner applies slow pressure just below the back of knee.

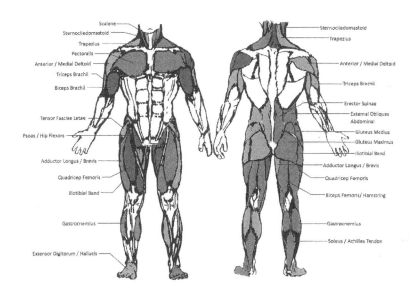

When these muscles shorten and tighten in response to the forces placed upon them, they fire poorly and in an uncoordinated fashion. Muscle testing a person's core muscles (abdominal muscles, erector muscles, quadratus lumborum and other core muscles), can show this type of compensation well. The side that is functionally superior more easily overcomes the practitioner and both the practitioner and the patient will be able to visualize the difference.

With overpronation, it is common to find muscular adhesion formation in the calf, anterior muscles of the leg, posterior muscle of the leg, and muscles in the back of the leg. A well-trained therapist can feel for the lesions that often create chronic pain and function, or acute muscle pulls with exertion. A well-trained health care practitioner knows the anatomy not only by what he learned in books, but by how it works as a chain of events. He understands how to both actively and non-actively evaluate the body.

Body style issues create certain mechanical compromises and these malfunctions can be reproduced on a patient to both confirm the practitioner's hypothesis based on the symptoms, history, body style and facts and predictably show these results to the patient. There is little guesswork and a high degree of predictability of what your health care practitioner should find using methods such as these. Providers who evaluate problems functionally can yield a higher level of reliability of diagnosis from practitioner to practitioner.

The concept of practitioner reliability is important because diagnosis in the musculoskeletal system varies widely from practitioner to practitioner. By using active evaluation, practitioners will see the problem the same way because it is diagnosed and named by function, not by symptoms; and it is seen as a mechanical problem, which it commonly is, rather than a symptom leading to a joint disease problem.

The pattern of test, treat, test in active evaluation methods shows real time improvement if the practitioner is performing an appropriate curative procedure. If not, there will be little change and the practitioner will then try different things during the treatment session until he sees muscular function and firing patterns improve about the area in question. This is why it is more cost effective than the typical diagnosis, manage the symptom with the same treatment for 10 visits hoping that at reevaluation time the person has improved. Our current insurance system does not allow for longer visits, which are sometimes desirable, for this process to be maximally effective.

An example of this is when I have a patient who is not having the desirable response after activity, and continues to have exacerbations. I have on occasion, on my own time (since the insurance carrier only pays for the relatively short visit) had patients stay in the office for an hour or two with the hope of finding the intervention that resolves a stubborn issue they are experiencing. I treat them, they run around the block once or twice or perform the task that continues to exacerbate the pain, they come back to the room, I evaluate them again, and continue to repeat this over and over, trying different interventions until the activity stops aggravating the problem. In many cases, this type of intensive test, treat and test using actual activities that cause the pain helps resolve the condition

In our current system of diagnosis when someone has pain in the left shoulder for example, one doctor may call it tendonitis, another may call it bursitis, another may call it a possible muscle tear, and another may call it an impingement syndrome. Then, following the flow charts and standard of practice for the area, doctors order higher-level expensive tests such as MRI after plain x-rays fail to confirm their suspicions. Many of these tests come back negative because their current level of analysis gives the practitioner an unclear way of truly seeing the mechanical basis of your problem.

Our schools teach practitioners to name the condition after performing standard tests to the area of pain; and then apply treatment to the named condition, often with little understanding of the mechanism behind what they are treating. Most practitioners have confidence in what they do to evaluate the problem because they learned it in a 'scientifically-based' educational institution. In the real world, this leads to frustratingly mediocre outcomes in rehabilitation, unnecessary drugs and surgery in our desperation to get relief.

> We have literally trained both the population and physicians to consider life-threatening conditions when symptoms occur as if they are a day-to-day occurrence.

Recently, a 16-year-old girl suffering from back pain came to see me. Her problem began 1 1/2 years earlier after playing basketball. She is 5'9" and experienced an extreme growth spurt a few years back. At first, she visited her high school athletic trainer who applied muscle stimulation (stimulating the muscles with measured electric impulses). She then visited her pediatrician who decided to send her for physical therapy when the patient's knees began to hurt.

The physical therapy helped her knees somewhat, but she had difficulty running. Her pediatrician then sent for bone scans and other tests and *then* her mother called our office after receiving our name from the high school trainer.

Upon initial questioning, I already knew by the complaints she volunteered that she had a foot problem. She had purchased off the shelf foot orthotics from the local running store, which helped.

Before she told me, I also knew that her neck was always tight and that she was having problems with the high jump (she does track and field and does not like running).

Evaluation showed torsion of the pelvis, tight and dysfunctional core muscles, tight hamstrings and limited neck and lower back motion. Visually, you could not help but notice the way she held herself as she stood in the exam room, with her one hip quite higher and the shoulders being rolled forward, more prominent on one side than the other.

Why couldn't one professional, preferably her primary care provider, look at her and see the whole picture? A more knowledgeable evaluator could have saved this child and her mom many doctor and therapist visits had they really understood what they were looking at. Incidentally, there were numerous opportunities for her pediatrician and others to identify her problems. Upon further questioning, this young girl told me she has always felt stiffness in her legs, back and neck.

I worked on her and she quickly improved and returned to her activities symptom free, while improving her ability to run and high jump. Running became more fun because she no longer had to endure pain to participate in the sport.

This patient's story is just one of many. This young girl's saga should help solidify for you the connection between body style, adaptation, why her back was hurting in the first place and why it is important to find an enlightened healthcare practitioner.

Myths, Facts and Consumer Cures

As previously stated, we adapt to stiffness and tightness that has been with us as we develop and grow except when it does not go away, or suddenly becomes very painful. We learn to take medication from our parents who learned it from their parents, or the media, or our doctors and we get worried when the problem does not go away anymore.

When a person sees her lifestyle affected, she seeks help from a health care provider she believes can help her. In the interim, she may avoid painful activities (Pain Avoidance behaviors), or take some over-the-counter or prescribed pain medication. The doctor often tells her to return if the pain does not go away or if it returns. The health care provider also adds a dose of comfort, reassuring her that her problem is not life threatening or orders her tests if there is a belief that something is not normal.

We have literally trained both the population and physicians to consider life-threatening conditions when symptoms occur as if they are a day-to-day occurrence. The truth is that life-threatening conditions happen infrequently.

The reality is that many people have mechanical problems. Mechanical problems that their first contact health care provider in the medical community often is not trained to evaluate properly because the problem mimics many internal disorders medical providers are most comfortable with evaluating. This is a major cost driver in our health care system.

Think about it for a minute… You have a pain. You get scared because it does not go away on its own. You go to your doctor who does not fully understand the problem, other than "it may be life threatening." Blood work-ups and other tests are ordered. Your doctor refers you to a specialist, who likely gives you a medication. You may also endure further workups for the condition depending on the disease state your health provider is attempting to rule out from his perspective. And there you are, no closer to a solution with the costs adding up quickly. There is a better way.

Evaluation of the musculoskeletal components would not only help many people get relief, but also improve the quality of their lives because many of these problems cause damage to the body joints over the years as they are ignored. Since the musculoskeletal system comprises over 50% of the body, it deserves equal attention and is usually the cause when medical tests are negative. Since medical tests usually come back negative, evaluation of the musculoskeletal system must be part of any workup by any healthcare provider for the care to be appropriate and cost effective.

Musculoskeletal conditions are *quality of life* threatening. These types of problems rarely considered first, as tests for life threatening illness have priority in our health care paradigm. Yet, problems in the musculoskeletal system are much more common.

It Stopped Hurting! Isn't That A Good Thing?

If the pain you had finally went away by itself, you would likely consider the problem to be self-limiting (self-resolving). Doctors think the same way.

The problem is that the mechanical cause of your pain still exists. It has likely become sub acute (minimally or non-painful with some occasional symptoms).

The mythic belief that painful problems just self-resolve with rest, and hurts only with certain activities is likely the reason many people have chronic pain that worsens with age. Typically, you avoid those activities that appear to aggravate the problem. You learn to use home or self-remedies such as ice, heat, pain relieving ointments or braces, believing they help when in fact; many braces just limit or change motion and pain relieving methods just relieve, and do not fix problem, which create the pain.

Over time, poor function damages the joints, tightens the muscles and often shows up years later as osteoarthritis. Since osteoarthritis develops over time, usually from increased stress and excess wear on an area, the arthritis on the films the doctor took is not the problem. Rather, it is a history of problem development.

When the degeneration becomes severe enough to impinge on nerves and irritate structures, it can then be discussed reliably as a causative reason for symptoms; but just because a joint shows wear and tear, it should not be assumed to be the cause of the damage.

Restricting your movement to avoid the pain creates a bigger problem. Studies show that exercise does not damage joints [82, 83]. Movement lubricates them with synovial fluid (joint lubrication).

Typically, most people respond to painful foot problems as follows...

1. You experience foot or heel pain.

2. You go to your drug store and get a heel cup to soften the blow on the heel. (There are many readily available products made to satisfy this need.)

3. You feel this is a solution because you experience less pain with the cushion. (Of course, without the heel cushion, you still get pain).

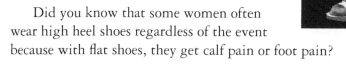

4. You may get an off-the-shelf foot orthotic that makes the foot feel better and less painful.

Did you know that some women often wear high heel shoes regardless of the event because with flat shoes, they get calf pain or foot pain?

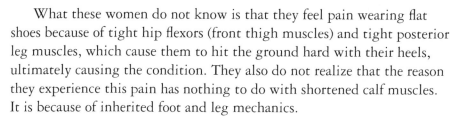

What these women do not know is that they feel pain wearing flat shoes because of tight hip flexors (front thigh muscles) and tight posterior leg muscles, which cause them to hit the ground hard with their heels, ultimately causing the condition. They also do not realize that the reason they experience this pain has nothing to do with shortened calf muscles. It is because of inherited foot and leg mechanics.

Do you want to know why wearing high heels feels better? Since she cannot turn her feet out in high heel shoes, wearing high heels minimizes her body asymmetry. It is like wearing Italian fashion-designer foot orthotics! Except, the more you wear the high heels, the shorter and tighter the muscles become creating an acute injury just waiting-to-happen.

As we try desperately to explore these self-made solutions, the problem gets worse as we age. It gets worse because we were ignoring the cause, believing the cause was the pain, which is a myth. Suddenly, we are older and out of ideas and now look for solutions that are more drastic because it hurts when we run or walk stairs. Our shoulder hurts when we reach or throw a ball with our son. We consider moving our upstairs bedroom downstairs because we cannot tolerate stairs due to knee pain. We stop going to the mall or the park because our ankle or foot hurts when we walk or, we get elbow or wrist pain when writing or typing a letter to a favorite aunt.

As we get older, we are told that we need more drastic measures like surgery, as the joints are inevitably damaged over time. We enter our golden years with chronic pain because the surgeries are designed to relieve the symptoms at the area of pain, not address the mechanical cause of the pain.

Gender-related knee problems are a great example. Many girls have damaged cruciate ligaments in their knees just from the simple and enjoyable act of jumping. This happens because many girls develop wider hips at puberty, which increases the greater angle at the knee (less stable and more likely to fail under extreme stress). Historically the problem is addressed with surgery. All better, right? Wrong. Here's why...

> A local hospital has been running ads for their department of orthopedics as if damaged cruciate ligaments in girls knees are normal.
>
> Two sisters tell about how one damaged the cruciate ligament in their right knee, then their left, and then the other did the same. It is so wonderful that this orthopedic department can fix what we may have been able to prevent had we screened these developing children properly in the first place.

The surgeon did not *fix* anything. He temporarily addressed the pain. The girl still has the same stress on her knees that initially created the problem!

Nevertheless, there is hope. Recently, athletic trainers have been learning about a program that strengthens core muscles which in turn decreases stress on the knees. The net effect is fewer cruciate injuries to girls.

We surgically implant replacement parts as the originals wear out due to improperly diagnosed body style issues and then, we box ourselves into the corner by only allowing activities that do not exacerbate the pain (known as pain avoidance behavior). Of course, the replacement joints never work like the originals and this negatively affects your quality of life.

Over time, this common approach, which we have been taught to believe is part of normal aging, causes inevitable consequences and unfortunately, our current health care model continues to encourage this poor behavior, making people suffer with pain as they age and adding billions on to the cost of health care in our country. Is it any wonder the cost of health care continues to explode as the population ages?

Simply put, we need a more appropriate model of health care. One that is more effective, costs less, and maintains the integrity of the body. This would result in greater activity, less pain and ultimately a better quality of life.

Insurance companies must not practice cost containment as the only way to keep costs in line, but steer people toward better behavior and help influence better lifestyles.

Currently, most have input solely from the medical groups infused with the current ideology that has tricked our drugged society into believing things just happen; a society that takes little ownership in its own health.

Our government is part of the problem, continuing to subsidize the production of foods that are not good for us such as corn sweeteners rather than subsidizing producers to grow nutritious food for a healthier public.

Insurance companies must show leadership and invite new ideas to sit at the table when they create policy.

Frustrating, isn't it? So, Fix it.

If you feel like your body is breaking down more and more as you age, and you stay away from activities because your body just doesn't tolerate it anymore without being in pain, you are experiencing the result of the difficulties with the current health care paradigm.

Even though your problem is likely a simple functional problem, it is just as likely that you have been to specialists. Specialists who recommended a few treatments, perform diagnostic tests, inject you with something or suggested you may have a problem that may require surgery as they try to find the 'itis', the 'opathy', or any number of horrible medical terms that can lead to more diagnostics and more high powered specialists.

You may have found the solutions offered only temporary relief. You may have been placed on medication that made you drowsy or nauseous and relieved your pain for short while. In the worst case, you had a procedure done after you were led to believe you had exhausted all your options and may have additional problems caused by the procedure.

Many people finally burn out when a problem is not resolved, a form of 'shell-shock" adding to their problems. In the patient's mind, nothing really worked and he guesses he is just getting older and has to live with it. Sometimes he goes further, with further interventions and scarier procedures, which can make him much worse off than before. His health care provider may even be convinced that his pain problem is psychosomatic and tell him, "What do you expect, you are getting older." Believe it or not, patients of mine were told this by their primary care doctors.

If that doesn't send you over the edge, you may have had the experience of visiting a managed care plan participating specialist and being cut off even though your improvement is steady but slow, as is the case working to improve function with many chronic problems that take time to improve and resolve. Managed care, as many discover, can be purely based on how little they can pay your health care provider, limiting the visits allowed and managing to the symptom. When your symptoms are gone (not when function is restored), you are disallowed the care you still need. The insurance company only covers acute conditions as a matter of policy, among other exclusions. Your potentially underpaid doctor shortens your visits, because the insurance company continues to squeeze him financially, making it unprofitable to spend the time to fully explore and fully figure out your problem. The 10 or 15-minute model of office visits will not work for everyone.

When the symptoms return because the problem was not resolved, it is an exacerbation or a new condition. If it happens too frequently, it becomes not medically necessary because the problem is not considered curable or the care given is not curative, a big problem with the disease/symptom model. I have had patients denied care or arbitrarily cut off from their needed care plan because the insurance company picked an arbitrary number of visits and decided not to pay anymore even though the care was curative and medically necessary.

In other words, in managed care, pain is the deciding factor for medically necessary treatment. Unfortunately, as you have learned, a lack of pain does not mean your body functions well. Here is how it translates in the current world: If your health care provider tests an area (knee, shoulder) and it does not function well against resistance, but it is not painful with normal activities, it is generally-considered non-clinical and care is not considered medically necessary to treat. The poorly functioning area will eventually become painful when you load it up playing basketball, tennis or do another activity. Treatment then becomes medically necessary (even though your provider may have prevented the problem from occurring with a minimal care recommendation) and you are fed into the medication- rehabilitation- surgery- medication-rehabilitation health care circle of hell at a much higher cost than if we acted before the symptoms presented themselves.

When performing a proper functional evaluation of the human frame, many areas that will become painful with activity are revealed. They show up during functional testing done by hand and without special and expensive blood tests or machines. Although you may not experience pain during your normal activities, functionally inadequate areas are painful when tested.

> You blame your pain on an activity, even though **you had the problem before you ever did the activity.**

Have you ever performed an activity that caused you pain where you believed that the activity was the cause? Many of us have. We blame it on the activity, without ever realizing we had a problem before we did the activity.

Most healthcare providers typically assume these pains to be symptoms of overuse-related injuries. Most doctors were just never taught to understand it from a functional point of view. It is like standing on a wood board that cannot support your weight. It looks like it can support your weight right up to the point where it snaps in two. We simply do not believe something is wrong unless it hurts. The reality is that the wood board can hold your weight right up to the point when it cannot.

This is why the disease-symptom paradigm we currently use often is misleading and results in many unnecessary and expensive tests when evaluating why someone is in pain.

Take note reader, it is the way your body functions mechanically that results in the process of most chronic back, neck, shoulder and joint pain.

Still don't believe me?

The other day I had a new patient with severe pain in her left shoulder and elbow. She could not even tolerate laying on it in bed.

First, she visited her primary doctor. I happen to know the provider personally and think he is thorough, open minded and a terrific internist. He referred her to a rheumatologist who immediately wanted to inject her shoulder with cortisone to alleviate the pain. Since the patient had a history of a problem with cortisone injection in her right foot treating plantar fasciitis a few years prior, she wanted another solution. During her evaluation, the rheumatologist also remarked that the patient had six tender points out of eighteen (how doctors currently diagnose Fibromyalgia) and suggested she was on her way to developing Fibromyalgia.

Thanks to the rheumatologist, now the patient was not only *still* in pain, but she was totally freaked out.

Panicked, she spoke with her primary doctor who referred her to me for the unenviable task of evaluating a scared and nervous patient. I explained to her that there might be other problems such a gait asymmetry since she had plantar fasciitis.

While taking her history I also found she could not turn her neck, a condition that is typical with tortipelvis, a distorted pelvis. During the evaluation, I confirmed that she indeed had tortipelvis, moderate to severe foot overpronation with the right side having more foot flare (foot turning out), and that her rib cage was shifted to the right causing severe straining of the rib heads on the left side of her shoulder blade.

On her first visit, I taped her feet into neutral (helping the leg work more effectively); resolved the distortion in her pelvis, and found entrapment of the supraspinatus muscle due to poor posture (this is the most common reason for non traumatic tears in the rotator cuff ; the muscles that control shoulder movement). The doctor's prescription was to go home, apply ice, and heat for relief.

On her second visit, she reported that she still could not tolerate lying on the painful shoulder. I moved her rib cage back into proper position and it stopped straining the rib heads on the shoulder eliminating the shoulder pain.

Her shoulder pain was resolved, but what about the elbow? After I performed the described manipulation, the elbow pain she experienced was immediately gone as well.

As you can see, a functional problem required a functional solution, based on a functional exam. I know she would not have had the same relief with a cortisone injection that left her body functioning poorly. The cortisone would have masked the pain, not corrected the problem.

> Researchers Janda and Singer pioneered active types of evaluation and published their findings specifically related to the effects of the leg on the spine and affiliated structures.
>
> **Physicians should read their findings.**

Body style is a determining factor of function period! A functional evaluation of these working parts is necessary to have a good understanding of why things do not work appropriately. The ability to evaluate the body in an active fashion is essential for the best results in treatment. The lack of knowledge about how the body works mechanically is the single most common reason for ineffective treatment and improper evaluation resulting in chronic pain, reliance on drugs for pain relief when therapy fails to succeed, long term joint damage and corrective surgeries that do not fix the problem.

While active evaluation methods in and of itself do not fix problems, it can be used to show you, the patient, a little about how your body works and why you get tight. It is also incredibly helpful for the health practitioner who is treating you, since he can visually see and feel how the body area in question reacts to the forces such as gravity and your normal daily tasks that are placed upon it. This knowledge is invaluable for people who suffer from chronic pain that no one has been able to help because they have an understanding of why they begin to tighten up and they understand their body style and its consequences. This leads people to be more knowledgeable about themselves and they armed with this knowledge can choose their style of caregiver more carefully.

Ankle Pain, Calf pain, Shin Pain and Knee Pain

Lower leg Pain is a common complaint handled in doctor offices. Calf cramps, ankle pains, knee pains and growing pains are frequently seen in primary care offices of internists, generalists and pediatricians. The first line of evaluation outside blunt trauma (having the knee or ankle injured by direct impact) is usually seeing your primary care giver (mandatory if you are in most HMO plans).

Typically, the doctor evaluates the area of pain and takes a patient history of how and when the pain began. The doctor explores the area, often performing some basic orthopedic tests (evaluation methods learned in school to help them diagnose and name the condition) and either gives you medication for the pain telling you to return if the pain continues, gives you self-care instructions or refers you for treatment to an orthopedic surgeon for further evaluation. At this point, you may have x-rays taken of the painful region or other diagnostic test such as an MRI; and then, if everything appears okay, get a referral for physical therapy directed at the area of complaint.

Is anybody reading this scenario shaking his or her head in agreement? Is it because this happened to you or a friend? Maybe it is because this is what you are used to seeing on television or experiencing yourself during a doctor visit for a pain or traumatic incident.

The major concerns for most people when they are sick are, "Do I have something life threatening?" or, "Did I do something wrong to make this happen?" Since health care practitioners want to avoid lawsuits if they miss a life-threatening event, in our litigious society, it is common for you to have multiple expensive tests done to protect them in case

> Conditions of this type merely consist of a series of symptoms and observations given a descriptive medical name, matched up with a treatment on a medical flow chart.

they miss something. This is especially true in emergency rooms, and is partly responsible for the high cost of those visits.

The problem is that the basics of musculoskeletal evaluation of the lower kinetic chain (ankle, knee, hip joints) are taught as separate conditions, rather than from a functional perspective. Many health care providers do not have a high level of confidence or certainty when they evaluate the lower kinetic chain, other than calling it a strain or a sprain.

An effective functional evaluation leads to a better experience and a more effective treatment of the cause of the problem. A non-functional evaluation is more likely to lead to the cause of the problem continuing to exist even when the symptoms may temporarily subside.

Often, a well-performed functional evaluation and sensible treatment path, even in an emergency, reduces the need for expensive tests. When we perform the proper care, most people improve eliminating the need for expensive high technology tests such as MRI whose over-sensitivity may lead to unneeded aggressive interventions and unintended consequences.

I live this example when I attend an athletic even as the medical director of New Jersey U.S.A. Track and Field and must perform on-the-field evaluations. Aside from my bag, some tape, a stethoscope and some other tools, I must take a history, evaluate the patient and create an intelligent course of treatment that will return the athlete to their event. Sometimes I can, and other times, if the injury is bad enough, I send the athlete to the emergency room. In my experience, more often than not, I can send them back to their event without a problem. Evaluation skills are essential for the musculoskeletal system.

The current system provides doctors little incentive to change; and there is great financial incentive for practitioners to not change. Some own imaging centers. Others have invested in surgical centers which are highly profitable because of ridiculous facility fees that are often far greater than what your doctor would earn for performing the procedure. This offsets the low fees they receive in most managed care plans. Health care has become one big game and the patients are caught in the middle.

There is, however, a small group of newer, more progressive practitioners learning active evaluation, which yields better information about what has malfunctioned in the myofascial system. The problem you have as a consumer is finding one of these rare, modern doctors. These doctors are practitioners of cause, not symptoms, and these are the people who are more likely to help you cost effectively.

My definition of a satisfactory outcome, one you should adopt, is one that improves the symptoms by improving the underlying cause of the problem and offers a good long-term improvement of function and freedom from symptoms in a reasonable period-of-time with a sensible cost structure.

In other words, the symptoms and problem should not merely feel better, but you should function better, without the need for medication for pain relief. You should be able to do more, tolerate more with less pain, and not feel like, "If I do this, it will begin to hurt all over again. Therefore, I will avoid that activity."

Feeling this way is pain avoidance behavior, and what I call "boxing ourselves into a corner." An acceptable outcome is an overall improvement in your quality of life and an improvement in the way you function without the threat of a recurrence during normal activities, especially as you age.

You do not have to avoid certain activities fearing recurrence of pain. It is not because you are older and you have to slow down. It is because someone has not adequately identified why you are in pain in the first place; and has not given you direction to resolve or significantly improve the overall problem.

Remember, the solutions to these types of problems are not found in a bottle, an injection, a splint or by avoiding the activity. Real solutions require looking outside the symptom box and evaluating how you are built, how your body works, and finding health care practitioners who can help you understand what you can do to make it work better.

Back pain

Most often, back pain is due to an asymmetry of the structures surrounding the pelvis. When one side is tight, the other side strains as the body attempts its normal movements. This is because each joint in the pelvis by design tolerates a certain amount of normal motion through the sacroiliac joints, hip joints and lumbar spinal joints.

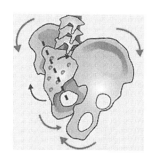

Asymmetry happens because of muscular imbalances and joint shape irregularities due to the way we walk, our foot posture and other body style inherited traits. A foot that toes out results in a knee that rolls in, which affects a hip that drops and rolls in causing excess forces through the pelvis. This torque on one side of the body causes the other side to compensate, straining the sacroiliac joints.

Since at least 50 percent of our body motion takes place through the pelvic joints, the torque locks up the pelvis, which causes the spinal joints to move excessively causing creep (a distortion of disc and joint fibers) that often leads to degeneration and tissue failure (a herniated disc or damaged disc fibers).

The shoulder on the same side of the foot flare will roll in, causing the muscles to tighten in response, the rib cage to rotate forward and the shoulder to dysfunction. This eventually tightens the muscles in the shoulder blade and neck on that same side because of muscular

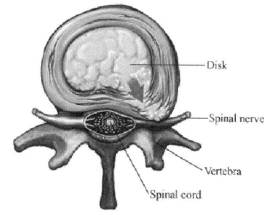

Disk

Spinal nerve

Vertebra

Spinal cord

recruitment (muscles that are firing inappropriate helping the body to maintain its mechanics despite poor leverage)[56].

Experience has shown that the person is most likely to feel the pain and sense tightness on the opposite side of the problem area (the side of the joint strain. This explains why back pain and its causes must be diagnosed correctly requiring your health care practitioner to look beyond the obvious symptom of pain and other symptoms. Merely looking at just the back pain and ignoring the rest of the body is why so many people suffer from multiple painful problems that come and go as they age. Managing each symptom as if it is different causes future problems, causing the explosion of aging people requiring hip and knee replacements. This is an industry based on diagnostic ignorance and a failure to preventatively screen and inform those who are biomechanically at risk.

Since most medical providers are trained to evaluate the symptoms, and our gut instinct as patients is to push doctors to find out what it is that is causing the back pain, the doctor, because of their limited understanding runs tests that most people do not need. A large portion of the populace has herniated discs in their spine that do not cause any symptoms; but when diagnosed during an episode, can become the source of an unnecessary and ineffective intervention[57]. In the end, the patient spends time and money on rehabilitation and other cures directed at symptoms without a reasonably predictable outcome because the true cause is unintentionally ignored. Many people have experienced Failed Back Surgery Syndrome over the years because of this.[58]

As a health care professional, I began questioning why doctor recommendations and patient results for treating pain are so unpredictable in the early 1990's. When I learned Active Release Techniques® (a registered diagnostic system of performing a style of myofascial release treatment) and started learning more about track and field and running injuries, I realized there was a disconnect in what I was learning and the causes of the problems I was seeing.

I remember asking Dr. Leahy, the founder of Active Release Techniques®, about the effects of foot overpronation on the process of scar tissue formation.

Although Dr. Leahy wrote about it in his thesis of the cumulative injury cycle (his explanation of why people who performed repetitive tasks had neurologic entrapment often diagnosed as carpal tunnel syndrome), at the time his theories and application was primarily aimed at the muscles, and how to find the lesions and treat them. At that time, during the mid 1990's, he was working to map the symptom to the malfunction in a systematic fashion, and then use his methods to resolve the complaint. He was designing pain charts to make it easy for doctors to succeed in treating those dysfunctions. I believed there was more to this model that needed to be uncovered and I was determined to find a way to make it easier to understand the feet, the application of foot orthotics and to perhaps, be able to create a reliable and easier way to create the rationale for using myofascial release and other styles of myofascial treatment.

I reviewed Dr. Brian Rothbart's bio-implosion model. His findings started increasingly making sense to me as more and more people visited our office with back pain and other joint-related complaints. With each patient I treated, I saw his model as an accurate depiction of what happens when body style responds to gravity. After evaluating thousands of patients, I am completely satisfied that the Rothbart bio-implosion model is a true predictor of the way a person's body compensates to the way they stand and walk. You will read and see more of Rothbart's work later in the "Body Mechanics" chapter of this book.

The literature is clear. We inherit major body features, including the way we walk and the way we are built, facial features, our height, the way we hold ourselves, and the predilection of possibly acquiring certain cancers or diseases.

It's no wonder entire families are surrounded by people in pain who believe it is normal because many of those surrounding them as they grew up had the same problems as they got older. Making matters worse, doctors regularly tell older patients that it is normal for their bodies to have these problems. This reinforces the "aging myth," in effect, causing disability and pain as people age and decreasing an individual's quality of life.

However, with the great majority of people, if we screen early for these problems and educate people how to take care of their body type, we can most likely get their body joints to last a lifetime allowing more people to enjoy healthy, active lifestyles with less pain, without disability, and without costly medical intervention.

Unfortunately, one of the major cost drivers for patient care is short sightedness of the caregiver and of the health care provider who did the original workup and referral. A physician is quite careful to avoid missing anything interpreted as negligence in today's litigious society. Teaching physicians to look at something, a certain way causes them to see everything that way....

Physicians are judged by community standards (performing as any other physician would perform in the same situation). As long as the physician is within the standard of care of his profession, and acted prudently, as other physicians in his geographical area would act, he is not negligent in the event of a poor outcome in the realm of musculoskeletal medicine. The standard of care may be wrong; however; if this is what his peers do, he has not violated public trust and is appropriate in your care, regardless of whether that care is mechanically appropriate for the condition. This is perhaps, why most doctors who have been party to failed back surgery syndrome by treating the symptom rather than the cause are not successfully sued for malpractice. They have not violated community standards!

Do you want to feel better? Find a doctor who has had someone show him a different and improved way to evaluate patients to add to his diagnostic tool kit.

During their initial visit to our office, most patients say they became aware of

An enlightened health care practitioner evaluates everything and is not blinded by his own or a patient's bias.

their problem when they performed a particular activity. They are often able to give me either an approximate or an exact date they believe the problem started. They stick by their story because to them, that activity is why they are in pain. Their current complaint became real to them the day it began hurting and disrupting their normal daily activities.

An enlightened health care practitioner evaluates everything and is not blinded by a patient's bias, but instead uses it as part of their complete history.

I have learned to encourage people to tell me about seemingly insignificant or unrelated problems that have come and gone. Often, these unimportant facts build me a road map, allowing me to solve their problem or point me toward what to look at to help them get out of pain. For this reason, I urge you to tell your health care provider everything, even when he does not want to hear those details.

I also urge you to convince your health care provider to check your feet, and pelvis as well as the symptomatic areas. Never assume that the symptomatic parts are the likely cause, especially if the problem presented itself over time and was not due to trauma. Moreover, if your doctor dismisses the idea, I urge you to find another doctor.

A health care practitioner who truly understands the musculoskeletal system and the kinetic chains will always consider the feet and pelvis. Until we reposition health care providers to take care of the causes of problems within the musculoskeletal system rather than obsess about the symptoms, many people will continue to suffer from chronic pain and require joints replacement after experiencing abnormal wear and tear.

This can only happen if our institutions of learning teach function rather than conditions, and introduce logical thought processes based on flow charts of function, rather than flow charts biased by the symptom model, which often leads to surgeries and more invasive methods of treatment. Furthermore, this can only happen if we as a society embrace the idea that many chronically painful problems people experience often is preventable by understanding function, and treating the mechanisms behind the pain, rather than attempting to manage only pain.

This prevention may include scoliosis *and* foot screenings while the children are in school. Remember, the army has done this to great effect, screening millions of soldiers for foot problems. Regulation 40-501 available online at http://www.army.mil/usapa/epubs/pdf/r40_501.pdf.

It may include evaluating feet and posture during the annual physical. It may include many specialists who deal with organ systems learning the interconnection between the human frame, organic disease and musculoskeletal conditions that can imitate many conditions like gastric reflux.

Many people suffering with a variety of symptoms go for invasive exams that might not be necessary if the health care provider understood how to evaluate the musculoskeletal system and that the musculoskeletal system needs to be a part of their regular diagnostic workup.

A treatment for mechanical pain will only be correct if it counteracts the mechanical dysfunction that ultimately created the problem. Telling someone who is in pain that it is likely arthritis after the medication failed to relieve the problem is not only unscientific, but it is harming millions of people who suffer the consequences of a lack of knowledgeable direction, education and treatment. This is a huge part of our explosive rise in healthcare costs as the population ages.

Many doctors still have a bias toward intervention and procedures. This partially is due to a system biased with hospital and procedure-based care during their hospital training and light on alternative not invasive methods by complementary health care providers. The financial incentives for performing procedures are much higher than doing evaluations and actual physical treatment to resolve the mechanical issue. This is why perhaps, most medical physiatrists do more invasive procedures, rather than actual treatment on their patients; it pays better.

The currently taught medical point of view is too narrow in scope. Over time, we can only hope this changes as the practice of health care continues to evolve.

Currently available solutions to manage many of the otherwise diagnosed conditions like Fibromyalgia, Carpal Tunnel Syndrome, joint replacement and surgeries include much better options and non-invasive methods. These include myofascial release, in particular Active Release Techniques (a style of myofascial release treatment that developed a reputation specifically for the way it handles carpal tunnel/cumulative trauma issues) and Graston Technique that uses specifically designed tools to restore tissue flexibility and break adhesion formation. There are other integrative schools of thought too, such as what Warren Hammer DC. DACBO is teaching in his Fascial Workshops ©.

Recently, doctors intrigued by research that shows that joint pain and the myofascial system are inseparable are taking the myofascial system much

According to the Bureau of Labor Statistics, U.S. Department of Labor, Occupational Outlook Handbook, 2010-11 Edition, `Physicians and Surgeons, on the Internet at http://www.bls.gov/oco/ocos074.htm (visited October 07, 2010) there are 661,400 Physicians and Surgeons and 49,100 Chiropractors in the U.S. comprised of:

- Allergists and Immunologists
- Anesthesiologists
- Dermatologists
- Family and General Practitioners
- Hospitalists
- Internists, General
- Neurologists
- Nuclear Medicine Physicians
- Obstetricians and Gynecologists
- Ophthalmologists
- Pathologists
- Pediatricians, General
- Physical Medicine and Rehabilitation Physicians
- Physicians and Surgeons, All Other
- Preventive Medicine Physicians
- Psychiatrists
- Radiologists
- Sports Medicine Physicians
- Surgeons
- Urologists

more seriously. Many musculoskeletal complaints result in or imitate internal organ complaints and disease processes because of the integration with the endocrine system. The recent acknowledgement that all these systems are in fact related puts our current system of treating different complaints as if they exist on their own into question.

Currently, we are overspecialized with organ and system based specialists. Excuse the cliché, but you cannot swing a dead cat without hitting a specialist focused only on his own discipline and the associated 'part' without consideration of the role the frame and musculoskeletal system plays in your health.

However, the rest of us know that in the real world, the body really is the sum of its parts. Both Myofascial Release and Graston have published studies, records of accomplishment with reliable results and have proven cost effective. They are methods of treatment that both professional and competitive amateur athletes find very reliable, very effective and very safe and as a result are in high demand. You can read case studies, research studies, patient testimonials and generally learn more about them at www.myofascialrelease.com and www.grastontechnique.com.

Unfortunately, only small portions of the medical establishment are familiar with them and do not regularly seek out providers specializing in the high quality delivery of these methods.

Choosing the Ultimate Health Care Team

The question many people have is, "Who should be on my health care team."

For most of us, it consists of a pediatrician and a primary care provider. We usually have a Dentist. A woman has a gynecologist who sometimes is listed as the primary care physician. In addition, more families are utilizing a family Chiropractor.

These providers are primary contact physicians and are the gateway to parts of our health care system. Most primary care physicians are not comfortable with evaluating the musculoskeletal system. They will refer these cases out for evaluation and possibly treatment. They will however, feel most comfortable prescribing medication that offers temporary relief and then refer you to a more appropriate health care provider.

Most dentists will evaluate you for tooth and gum related problems, and refer you to other specialists who deal with gums, periodontal work and other dental sub-specialists.

A pediatrician is the primary care provider for developing children. Pediatricians also take care of initial vaccinations and act as archivists of medical record information needed for camp, preschool and societies other requirements. Like most primary care providers, however rarely, they refer out most musculoskeletal problems because they do not treat these conditions. They do however, evaluate and then refer them to an appropriate provider.

Many more families do now use chiropractors who are very comfortable with the musculoskeletal system and also are able to treat many conditions of the spine and extremities effectively without the use of medications. Unfortunately, many people find the chiropractor on their own after experiencing utter disappointment with their current medical care. More primary care providers are now making chiropractic referrals and establishing referral relationships with those they trust. The Annals of Internal Medicine in 2007 introduced guidelines for this[26].

Internal organ and disease related problems worked up by primary care doctors are often connected to the musculoskeletal system. Few medical specialists consider this in their manual evaluation resulting in many tests that are often inconclusive, costing the patient, the insurance company and the health care system in general millions of dollars annually.

If most medical specialists had a better understanding of the musculoskeletal system their evaluation, would likely include fewer upper and lower GI tests, fewer MRI tests and X-rays, and other tests that could b e eliminated by better evaluation skills. This can help lead to more appropriate referrals and better long-term outcomes.

The Health Care Team For Your Body Should Include:

 A Chiropractor

At the risk of offending your sensibility, I understand this sounds predictable and self-serving. Nonetheless, some of the most brilliant health care providers of the musculoskeletal system I know are chiropractors.

More doctors are not only referring to chiropractors but are also using them as well. Back pain in the surgical suite is a common complaint of medical specialists who are beginning to embrace the value of the chiropractic profession for themselves. It makes sense. Surgeons, doctors and nurses stand on their feet all day long, subjecting their skeletal and muscular frame to the ravages of gravity.

Chiropractic is the profession most noted for manipulation of the spine (care of the human frame) and has the most experience performing the procedure. Spinal manipulation is also proven safe and effective, with chiropractic doctors having some of the lowest malpractice insurance in the health care industry.

Chiropractic is holistic in nature and is the only profession in the United States that attempts to fully understand the care of the human frame by caring for the spinal joints and the extremities.

Since chiropractors do not rely on drugs or surgery, they concentrate on non-invasive, conservative care methods while using the skill of spinal and extremity manipulation to get the results people have come to expect.

Current trends in chiropractic care are moving away from passive care like heat, muscle stimulators, ultrasound, and other machines, and moving toward hands on treatments such as Myofascial Release, Graston, Active Release Techniques®, Trigger Point and other myofascial treatment regimens. Current trends also include exercises that enhance the effect of these methods to improve long-term outcomes.

Foot Levelers, Inc., a company that manufactures custom-made, flexible orthotics based on chiropractic research and innovative technology called for chiropractors to check their patient's feet and gait for problems that can lead to problems in their frame and associated symptom complexes. Chiropractors who had not reached the same conclusion as I did regarding the impact that foot overpronation and gait have on a patient's health took up the company's challenge. Today, many chiropractic practitioners regularly do this as part of their initial evaluation.

Manipulation of the joints of the spine and extremities is vital to asymmetrical bodies because it works toward improving joint function and movement and helps reestablish better body symmetry as well as mobility. The idea of manipulation has been practiced for thousands of years (bonesetters) for good reason; it is cost effective and it works. Manipulation of the soft tissues (muscles, tendons and ligaments) is vital because this holds the human frame in place. As you cannot separate one from the other, most chiropractors work on both the soft tissues and the joints with manipulation type procedures.

Massage Therapist

Massage therapy is essential for a health muscular system. Of course, like chiropractors, different massage therapists have their own style. Moreover, those getting out of schools now have the latest skill set. Others participate in continuing education to stay ahead of the curve. These people should be part of your life. Some use Myofascial Release, Sports Massage, compressive techniques, hot rocks as well as other methods to relax tight dysfunctional muscles so the muscles can function more efficiently.

Many of the therapists I have visited use integrative techniques. This simply means they use a variety of techniques appropriate to the patient's need instead of sticking with one particular style. The right massage therapist can be quite helpful to you. A good massage therapist will know when and is willing to refer you out when they believe your problems are larger than they can handle with their methods.

Primary Care Physician (internist, family practice)

Your primary health care provider is like the quarterback in the health care system. He is in charge. Especially when you are ill and need to be admitted to the hospital for care. Some are medically trained and others, like the doctor I personally use is an Osteopath, whose heritage began more similarly to that of chiropractors with manipulation being their main tool. Over the years however, most Osteopaths work more like your local medical physician and no longer use manipulation. Other than the letters after their name, you will see little difference between medical and osteopathic primary care doctors.

Find a Primary Care doctor who is open to new ideas, is conservative in their approach and is cautious about latest medications. Remember, doctors are bombarded by information supplied by drug representatives that can influence their behavior on recommending drugs.

Your better physicians of any healthcare discipline will always question everything, including themselves and their decisions as they continue their years of practice. Your better physicians will council you when necessary, and not always rely on drugs as a remedy. Your better physicians will be open to many options for your care and are always continuing their education, looking to be either up to date with, or at the forefront of change in their professions.

If you are in an HMO and need a referral, your primary care physician should be ready to make the process easy and accommodating for you. You should be able to get an appointment quickly. If you have to wait when you get to the doctor's office, the visit should not be an all day affair due to excessive waiting times. You want to be confident that if you have a serious or life-threatening health problem they will make the process easy for you and have a staff caring enough to go the extra mile for you in that time of crisis.

If you are hospitalized, you want to feel confident your doctor is there for you making the right decisions regarding your stay in the facility. That can mean a fight with the hospital, referring you to health care providers you can trust and with whom you will feel comfortable; especially when requesting a particular in-network health care provider.

A rising trend is the Physician Extender. People are finding that their primary care doctor has a physician extender in the office. This can be a Nurse Practitioner or a Physician's Assistant. Doctors are employing these medical professionals so they can see more patients, more cost effectively. These are people trained to handle many common medical conditions.

You can also find nurse practitioners and physician's assistants in some places you don't naturally equate with medical health care... aside from picking up toothpaste and prescription drugs. Some quick clinics located in Walmart, CVS and other stores rely exclusively on these physician extenders and offer their medical services at a relatively inexpensive cost, while handling the 40 or more common uncomplicated conditions as they would in your local physician's office.

Perhaps, health care is becoming more convenient as this model of care becomes more common.

 ## Dermatologist

In this current age of sun over-exposed bodies, a good dermatologist can be indispensable. From warts, to skin cancers, early diagnosis is the most important thing that can happen. Your primary doctor, chiropractor or other physician may know of a good dermatologist and can be a source of a great referral for you. Always look for someone who can see you for an appointment within a reasonable period of time (within a week or two). A good dermatologist will be cost effective and have sharp diagnostic skills.

 ## Orthopedist

At times, we find ourselves with injuries to the musculoskeletal system that cannot be handled conservatively and require someone with the expertise to repair a broken limb or damaged joint. Orthopedists are surgeons who trained to help repair broken limbs and repair damaged joints. As surgeons, they evaluate and screen people to see if a surgical solution is appropriate for the area of complaint.

A good orthopedist will send anyone needing conservative care out for rehabilitation or a non-surgical intervention before recommending going under the knife. Few orthopedics refer patients to chiropractors and many view chiropractors as competitors. Frankly, that's silly and strictly speaking a selfish income-based decision. A chiropractor does not perform surgeries, so there is no competition there and a chiropractor needs a trust-worthy orthopedist to recommend when a patient's condition calls for it.

In offices where orthopedic doctors and chiropractors work together, the relationship is usually rewarding for both the doctors and you, the consumer who benefits from the collaboration. When choosing at orthopedist, find out how he feels about referring patients to non-surgical musculoskeletal, complementary medical solutions and providers.

Physical Therapist/ Occupational Therapist

This profession has its origins in World War II as a solution to help rehabilitate the wounded. Of course, like any health profession, it has evolved and they help treat many hospitalized people recovering from surgery, or who have loss of function of a limb or area of the body.

This hands-on profession is not typically a first contact provider and in most states requires a referral from your doctor, similar to other medical specialists.

Many larger practices can look like gyms and offer hands-on exercise instruction and therapy to reach the goals the referring doctor has set. Often, particularly with occupational therapy, sessions take place in the patient's home, or in a health care treatment facility. Most people who have had surgical repair to a limb, or a joint replacement meet with a physical therapist to help them become more limber and healthier.

These therapists commonly work with stroke victims, post-surgical rehabilitation and geriatric rehabilitation and of course, are engaged regularly for rehabilitation of the knees, hips, neck and back. Some take additional courses in manipulation realizing that chiropractors are the gold standard when it comes to spinal and extremity manipulation.

Section III

You

Understanding Your Pain

Why are results so incredibly erratic when treating your pain? Why is it that Bob, who sits in the cubicle next to you, seems fine while you struggle to get out of your chair for a trip to the water cooler?

Back and neck pain costs Americans more than 86 billion dollars annually in both lost work productivity and in lifestyle effects[1]. Millions undergo back treatment from numerous sources including physical therapists, chiropractors, physiatrists, pain management specialists, and rheumatologists. Still, treatment costs continue to skyrocket and we still do not truly understand "what is back pain"[2].

Here's why; Many problems in the neuromuscular system also present like internal disease processes. Yet our primary care physicians lack the training in manual evaluation skills and process to properly rule out the musculoskeletal system before giving you a shot, prescribing medication, and ordering tests to rule out disease processes[3].

This missing background in functional evaluation results in an over reliance of costly and invasive tests; leads to painful risk-laden interventions; and places many of us on medications, several of which have recently been removed from the market due to negative side effects[4] worse than the problems they were treating. Instead, shouldn't your doctor be able to find a better solution; One that is less invasive and typically much safer?

The Boston Globe and New York times on February 13, 2008 reported the following[59]:

> ## "NEW YORK - AMERICANS ARE SPENDING MORE MONEY THAN EVER TO TREAT SPINE PROBLEMS, BUT THEIR BACKS ARE NOT GETTING ANY BETTER.
>
> Those are the findings of a report in the Journal of the American Medical Association, which found that spending on spine treatments in the United States totaled nearly $86 billion in 2005, a rise of 65 percent from 1997, after adjusting for inflation.
>
> Even so, the proportion of people with impaired function because of spine problems increased during the period, even after controlling for an aging population."

Evidence continues to show that our current U.S. medical system's solutions have neither improved the problems associated with how we treat back pain, nor improved the quality and cost effectiveness of care.

If our health care providers do not change what they are doing and how they perceive conditions of the back, the neck and the balance of the skeletal system, they simply cannot expect patient results to improve. Moreover, as history shows, the costs will continue to uncontrollably spiral upward.

It is well past time to stop repeating our mistakes. It is time for real change. "Insanity is doing the same thing over and over and expecting a different outcome". Do we really need famed

Neuromuscular system: Relating to or affecting both nerves and muscle tissue

Disease symptom process: a condition not from physical injury resulting in pathological symptoms

Pathological symptoms: relating to or arising from a disease

Functional evaluation process: Test, challenge, treat, and repeat until the area in question improves functionally and measurably

theoretical physicist Albert Einstein to rise up from the grave and slap us silly to see that enough is enough?

Based on experience treating people with chronic symptoms for over twenty years, America's obsession with symptom diagnosis, instead of seeing the bigger picture functionally and understanding the systems that create pain and body breakdown has left many people in chronic pain looking for alternatives to the traditional health care approach of drugs, tests, exercises and surgeries.

Current studies show an increasing population is embracing alternative and complimentary health care providers to get relief beyond what the traditional health care systems paradigm is capable of offering[25].

Back pain, neck pain, joint pain, shoulder problems and many other painful conditions of the musculoskeletal system often fail to respond to treatment because the schools of traditional health care are teaching health care providers each condition is its own entity, rather than because of poor function of a system or systems.

Insurance company coding reinforces this thinking since every symptom must have a code, however, the codes describe the symptomatic part in many cases rather than the dysfunction that is causing the area to become symptomatic. Therefore, it is considered appropriate and common practice to direct a trial of care based on a symptomatic region. Nevertheless, this is wrong...

Fixing this problem requires we need a change in way doctors understand, evaluate and ultimately treat back pain and other conditions involving the spine and the affiliated structures that include the arms and legs.

The belief that different organs and joints are totally independent, with specialization in the treatment of the parts, instead of the whole is lunacy. This type of approach has proven to be expensive and inefficient. Patients invest time, effort and money trying to get relief looking for alternatives when the traditional piecemeal model does not solve their problem. This has lead to the steady rise of alternative and complimentary care providers who have different thought processes and often solutions that result in higher patient satisfaction in a growing industry that people are, in many cases, funding without insurance.

The musculoskeletal, the hormonal, and the neurological systems of the body connect through chemical, neurological and other pathways. Since systems of the body function interdependently, some in ways we have yet to understand fully, having specialists view symptoms as if they are the problem rather than understanding the malfunction in the systems does not really work. Our exploding healthcare costs are a symptom of this of this problem with today's faulty evaluation and treatment process.

Getting Help - Learn From Patient Case Studies

A patient I treated years ago was doing quite well and, as often happens, stopped visiting the office, even for periodic check-ups. After a seven-year absence, she scheduled an appointment, telling me about a number of health problems she had acquired, including diabetes.

While taking her history, this otherwise active woman immediately gave me a long list of medications she was taking regularly.

She was having lower back and neck problems that became severe enough to prompt a return to our office. Prior to her lower back, neck and shoulders becoming very painful, she had problems with her feet that were causing stress fractures which are typically due to inherited poor foot mechanics.

The patient spent two years wearing surgical boots, as her feet appeared to almost self-destruct with repeat fractures. Finally, after two years of torment, she was able to tolerate wearing sneakers.

At the time, her doctors had not considered referring her back to her chiropractor, but instead, preferred to send her for pain management.

She did not like some of the invasive recommendations and eventually called us.

> You can read about stress fractures online here:
>
> http://orthopedics. about.com/cs/ otherfractures/a/ stressfracture.htm

I re-evaluated her and found she badly needed orthotics (shoe arches). Her feet had an inherited trait that caused her to bear weight unevenly and ineffectively. Her foot type, being flat, wide and flaring out is prone to developing stress fractures because of the inefficient way it disperses stress as she walks or runs.

The patient was "prescribed" off-the-shelf arch supports. She reported they felt terrific and she noticed her lower and upper back immediately felt an improvement as well.

Within three visits providing chiropractic manipulation, arch supports, and myofascial treatment to her core muscles, her pain was markedly reduced and she was walking more normally.

Had she had her gait and structure evaluated early in the process, she could have avoided foot fractures, two years of painful walking in pair of orthopedic boots and the high personal and financial cost of this haphazard management of her problem. She was clearly heel striking quite hard on both sides due to the tightness in her legs.

It is more than likely she could have also avoided weeks of back and neck pain as well since these were clearly structural problems and needed a structural solution.

Unfortunately, many patients are lead astray by health care providers who do not understand how the musculoskeletal system integrates, into itself and into other organ systems. As a result, countless people have each symptom treated separately, with each 'solution' requiring 2-3 medications that load the patient up with drugs that mask the symptoms; sometimes creating life-threatening side effects with long term usage.

> **Structural problems need a structural solution.**

This is a costly and dangerous solution that does not address the main problem, which is clearly based on mechanical dysfunction. When we look at health care quality and the cost as people age, is it any wonder that our obsession with symptoms rather than function has had an expensive effect without a necessary improvement in the care people receive?

Preventing Surgical Procedures and Joint Replacements

A recent patient complained of lower back pain that began six weeks ago, followed by neck and shoulder pain a few weeks later – all before our visit.

He told me that his father has chronic lower back and disc problems, an important clue since body style traits are inherited.

The patient's prior history tells the story of how he began to have pain in his foot two years prior to seeing me. His orthopedist diagnosed a stress fracture in his foot and casted the foot. Soon after, the medial side of his knee began to hurt. The orthopedist put him on crutches and said he had a medial knee stress fracture. Then, his other foot started hurting. The patient was told he had a stress fracture in the other foot and needed to be in a wheelchair, which he refused to do.

Finally, in the patient's mind, these problems resolved. However, the problem never resolved, the symptoms merely subsided to the point he was able to minimally function.

During my evaluation, I noticed that he not only had very flat feet but that his feet also turned out, more on the right, which caused his pelvis to torque and distort. The orthopedist he visited never considered that his feet may be involved and took care of each symptom assuming they were from an overuse.

> **A later section discusses the process of stress fractures and why they occur in greater detail.**

The patient's problems then, and today, are a consequence of body style and faulty body mechanics. Since he was never functionally evaluated, he endured pain likely due to poor function rather than stress fractures. Typically, stress fractures are a *consequence* of how we use our bodies and pre-existing problems created by how we are built (body style).

I explained to the patient from a functional and mechanical perspective why he had the problems a few years ago, and why he currently experiences lower back pain. I also explained that he needed inserts in his shoes to help prevent further problems in the future.

It is highly likely that he had unrecognized symptoms prior to his visit to the orthopedist or this chiropractors office, but didn't know it; believing his issues to be normal since we establish our body styles at an early age and we accommodate to what we are familiar with.

Clearly, the management of this persons problems was inadequate because the symptoms, rather than the functional causes were addressed, causing him to suffer needlessly and endure complications that were avoidable.

This type of management often results in a higher cost of care, inconsistent results and patients who may drop out of care because they figure they just have to live with the problem after committing time and resources to ineffective diagnosis or treatment.

Back Pain Treatment, what is wrong with this picture?

I received a call in the office regarding a patient who was in horrible pain. She had heard about the Graston Technique®, a method my office uses in the treatment of the muscular and fascial structures to reduce pain and improve function.

The patient described her chronic pain journey.

For nearly a decade, she had seen doctor after doctor to treat her for painful hips, knees, back, shoulders. Eventually, she was advised that she needed a right-side hip replacement. Thinking that she finally had a solution to her problem, she had the replacement surgery performed.

After the surgery, the pain in her back and legs did not subside, nor did her limp. A few years after the hip replacement surgery, she was advised to have back surgery to treat the pain in her back and legs. She submitted to this surgery as well.

A few years after her back surgery, her limp became more noticeable and she was advised that her left hip now needed to be replaced and that her right knee, the one on the side of her original hip replacement was going bad.

She was also told that over the last two years, a significant difference in height developed between both hips and that the doctor would address this during the surgery per his measurements.

Again, she submitted to the surgery. Afterward, she could no longer stand for more than a minute or two without losing her balance or feeling pain.

Continuing to search for solutions, she read about the Graston Technique® as a non-invasive way help break down scar tissue and myofascial restrictions using instrument assisted soft-tissue mobilization treatment.

Not to be fooled again so easily, she wanted to try Graston Technique® before submitting to additional procedures at the discretion of a local physiatrist who strongly recommended epidural injections in her spine for pain relief.

At this point in listening to her story over the phone, I stopped her and commented, "It sounds like everyone is looking at your symptoms, but not at you."

I asked, "Has anyone evaluated the way you walk, the way you stand or the effect the last surgery had on your structure?"

"No.," she replied.

I then suggested that instead of discussing just one of the tools of the chiropractic trade that she come in and permit me to evaluate her.

While she was filling out the initial forms for her office visit, I looked over the inch-thick packet of surgical reports, justifications for procedures and the like.

Each specialist looked at her painful areas and ran their tests, which were limited to the regions of pain. Each specialist then gave her the bad news and the recommendation that surgery was necessary or she would live in pain forever, or lose her ability to sit comfortably, to drive, to walk, or even to stand.

In the specialists' minds, each area just went bad and needed fixing immediately. Ironically, her body was self-destructing, and becoming less functional with each attempt to fix the problem due to her and her doctor's actions.

My first concern was to make sense out of what was done, to put all the doctors in communication with one another and to coordinate both their care and their thought processes.

Unfortunately, when I called the physiatrists office, suggesting he contact me to discuss his direction, and thought process, the case was pulled from me.

He really must have wanted to give her an epidural injection. Maybe he was on a quota. Why else insist upon an epidural injection; a fashionable less conservative approach done frequently today that has only a 30% success rate at best, yet is commonly recommended as an effective solution[60].

Did the patient really need the epidural spinal injections and would it have truly benefitted her? The injection addresses a site of pain, rather than the mechanics that is creating the problem. How is the injection going to have the patient's body functioning better?

Could this entire scenario have been avoided with a better approach to this patient's problems?

Unfortunately, the significant damage was done before she ever stepped foot in my office and all I could do was damage control.

I have seen thousands of cases just like this. Hopefully, the thought process in this book will help us change the course of care that allows scenarios such as this one.

In my clinical experience, most patients and their physicians believe the pain is the problem and it needs treatment. In other words, your shoulder hurts; therefore, the problem is the shoulder.

You as the patient believe the doctor has the answers and is the one to help you ultimately feel better. However, many painful problems or syndromes are classified as diseases or degenerative processes rather than what they are: manifestations of poor mechanics, which for most people is something an enlightened practitioner can improve by thinking outside the box.

Most people falsely believe that these types of problems should self-resolve; or as I have often heard before, "work themselves out". ,

There is in fact always a reason or a basis for why something hurts. Symptoms often are not a reliable predictor of health, especially in the musculoskeletal system.

Moreover, as tremendous a resource as it is, the internet is not very helpful dispelling the current diagnosis belief, with websites that reinforce the symptom myth featuring "Symptom Checker" search engines. A trusted high profile example of this is Mayoclinic.com (http://mayoclinic.com/health/symptom-checker/DS00671).

Pain Basics – Knowledge is Power

Pain Avoidance Behavior vs. Finding a Solution

Over the years, I have met many people who decided that as they got older, their bodies could no longer tolerate certain activities. Some are as young as their thirties and forties.

Many people have visited health care providers only to assume that since nothing has helped them other than Advil®, or another pain reliever, their problems were unsolvable. As they aged, and they asked their regular doctors for better solutions, they often were told that it is normal for this to happen, as it is a part of aging.

Typically, these people slowly remove activities from their lifestyle they believe aggravate their problem. For instance, they may give up running because their knees or hips hurt. They may hang up their glove and give up softball because they increasingly experience injuries when running or throwing. They may avoid getting on the floor with their grandchildren because of soreness, or eliminate other activities like tennis as their joints hurt and they decide it is just not worth the pain and suffering of attempting to stay active.

This describes pain avoidance behavior, which is simply avoiding activities that appear to aggravate an existing problem or makes the person hurt.

I have treated hundreds of patients over the years that put themselves through this because they truly believed that as they got older, their body would cannot tolerate certain activities and they needed to "slow down". What they did not realize is that in their immediate families, people who not only looked like them, but who are also built like them surrounded them.

These people, in all likelihood, experience many of the same problems because they are built the same way.

A few people I treat take a different tact. I have some patients who do Pilates® training and the activity has actually helped their condition. However, since they cannot perform certain maneuvers without pain, the instructor modifies the activity so they can tolerate it. In the end, they are stronger, but the original problems are never corrected, creating the need for continued Pilates® classes. This is simply creating a stronger and physically fit *disabled* body.

I regularly meet with patients who religiously visit the gym 3-4 times weekly because this "keeps me feeling good." Upon carefully questioning most of them, what I find is that they go to the gym or martial arts training this frequently because they stiffen up with inactivity and sitting makes them ache in their lower back or in their shoulders and neck.

Since they feel good when working out, they make it a priority to work out continuously because they would feel terrible if they did not exercise.

One recent patient, an employee of Johnson and Johnson® near my office, visited us for a chronic lower back problem that became exacerbated.

Upon questioning her, I found out she worked out at least 3 times weekly to keep herself feeling good and keep out of pain. When I asked her what happens when she did not work out, she stated her lower back would be painful after sitting a while and her shoulders would be tight and painful. She believed the exercise helped her prevent the problem. However, this current episode made it impossible for her to work out. After a number of visits, which included working on her pelvis, neck, shoulders and legs, there was no longer any pain, even when sitting for long periods. She is back to working out, however now her motivation is to stay healthy and feel good, as opposed to pain avoidance.

There is a better way to treat problems such as these. In order to find that better way, you as a consumer must think about pain and function differently. Your health care providers must also look past the obvious as well. The symptom based approach to evaluation and treatment is largely responsible for people living like this. Imagine what life would be like without issues like these preventing you from doing what you love.

In my experience, the only limiting factor for people to improve at any age is the overall condition of the joints in your body. Even if the joints are arthritic, you can slow the degenerative processes markedly by doing the right thing; improving your body mechanics.

Rethink the idea that as you get older you should experience more pain. Eliminate the idea that osteoarthritis is a normal part of the aging process. Wear and tear is normal, but why do some people break down and have many more problems than others have. If we were all destined to have these problems, wouldn't we all be in pain as we age?

Even medical doctors that chiropractors treat believe the problem is arthritis. Is it any wonder most people think this way? Your body goes through changes in your 20's, 30, 40's, with the 40's **Example #2** being a transition for many people who never took care of themselves and now find that doing normal everyday things creates muscle aches, pulls and joint injuries. In other words, you cannot get away with what you got away with in your 20's and 30's without feeling it too much. Osteoarthritis is not necessarily present because you are old. It is an unpleasant fact if you are built asymmetrically.

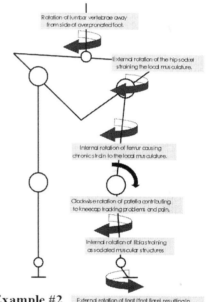

Rotation of lumbar vertebrae away from side of overpronated foot.

External rotation of the hip socket straining the local musculature.

Internal rotation of femur causing chronic strain to the local musculature.

Clockwise rotation of patella contributing to kneecap tracking problems and pain.

Internal rotation of tibia straining associated muscular structures.

External rotation of foot (foot flare) resulting in poor foot posture. The muscles overwork creating predictable pain patterns as you age.

This effect can really be accentuated by certain body styles; remember, not everyone is miserable after 40 and, since soft tissue trauma is cumulative, any injuries or accidents not properly attended to myofascially and joint-wise gets worse over time and creates long term damage to the spine and extremities.

Current evidence suggests that stiff hypo mobile (insufficiently mobile) joints degenerate at a faster rate than moving joints. By the age of 40, the discs in our back lose their moisture, which is one of the main reasons mechanical problems in the pelvis become more noticeable in the neck and back[61]. (www.healthscout.com, www.ehow.com.)

Another unpleasant fact is that if your body is build more efficiently and symmetrically, you are less likely to have severe chronic pain as you get older and your flexibility will be better compared to someone built with low or flat arches and asymmetry. Admittedly, this is good news for you. For the rest of us, it is just more bad news. We need to be smarter to have a healthier spine, pelvis, shoulders, knees and hips.

The good news is that for many years now, there have been methods to improve the way we stand, walk and function; and the great thing is, all you have to do is buy the right type of footwear, wear inserts in your shoes if needed and buy sandals with arches for walking around during the warmer weather.

Back Pain Basics – Kinetic Chains? What are they and what does this have to do with pain and stiffness?

In order to understand the underpinnings of lower back pain, or functional joint and muscular pain in the human body, you have to understand that the way we walk has much to do with problems you experience in your back, neck, affiliated spinal joints and extremities. Remember, we inherit certain traits and the likelihood of back pain is an inherited trait, based on the way we walk.

Humans are not the only ones who experience back pain and degeneration based on body style. People who own pets know for instance that certain breeds of dogs develop back problems and some breeds are prone to having arthritic hips. I bring this up because problems with gait are not exclusive to animals that stand upright, such as human beings. Race Horses have special shoe fitters who level out certain horses with special shoes so they race faster with fewer injuries.

The human body does not tolerate asymmetry well. The more asymmetrical you are built, the more likely you will experience lower back pain as well as sciatica, neck pain, hip pain, upper body pain including shoulder pain and neck pain

With all this talk about the effect your feet have on your health, you might be thinking, "Sure. Having flat feet is an issue. Everyone knows that." (http://www.aurorahealthcare.org/yourhealth/healthgate/getcontent.asp?URLhealthgate=%2296921.html%22; http://www.mayoclinic.com/health/flatfeet/DS00449.)

Are you ready for the truth? Having flat feet does not necessarily mean you will have back pain. Recent studies cannot prove conclusively that having flat feet creates back pain. The affect of foot flare on the body, however, and the affect of one foot turning out more than another does have an effect, when studied from an engineer's point of view[62].

If He Walks Like a Duck...

The feet are your body's foundation. When the foot turns out as you walk, the knee on that side rolls in. The net effect called a functional short leg really refers to the leg's position, and that the leg appears shorter. The more the foot toes out, the less efficiently you can walk and run. It also creates knock-knees and eventually causes damage to the inside of the knee. If you have ever seen someone who has the classic duck walk where both feet flare out noticeably, you will know what I mean.

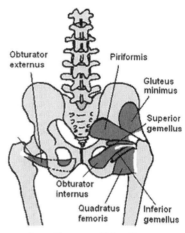

http://www.wikipedia.com

Toeing out aggravates classic overpronation sometimes known as fallen arches, which means the tibia (the shin bone) rotates in excessively as you walk, stressing the muscles in the ankle, the ankle joints and the muscles that attach to your shins, with secondary effects in the back and neck regions.

This is why people who walk this way often experience shin pain when they run without appropriate foot support. As they walk, internal rotation of the femur (thighbone) increases stress at the hip socket. This high stress and inefficient movement overstrains the joints beyond the force they were designed to tolerate. This results in arthritic knees, improperly tracking kneecaps, leg cramps, hip and back pain, as well as many conditions of the upper back, neck and shoulder and may even be a causative factor in idiopathic scoliosis, a curvature of the spine that occurs without an understood cause.

Another effect is the shortening and tightening of the gluteal and piriformis muscles (your buttocks and surrounding muscles), which can cause eventual problems with the sciatic nerve, the body's largest nerve trunk.

The hamstrings, the muscles on the back of the leg will also be tight on the same side. This is the beginning of potential problems because tight hamstrings and tight calves normally exist together as the person slams their foot into the ground as they walk. If this goes on long enough, they can get heel pain, or plantar fasciitis (pain on the tissues at the bottom of the feet called the plantar fascia).

Be aware of this the next time you are told the problem is just plantar fasciitis or a heel spur and the provider who diagnoses you only addresses the foot pain, and ignores the legs, pelvis and other areas that are inevitably part of the problem. Keep reading...

The side of foot flare effectively lowers the hip, which now causes shearing forces at the sacroiliac joints, the joints that hold the pelvis together. Meanwhile, the minor undulations that occur in the lower back joints, the vertebrae, become more exaggerated and can create a process called "creep" in the spinal discs that can cause disc fibers to initially distort, fail and create the classic acute lower back or sciatic syndrome when someone bends over to do something. Then the back goes out or locks up leaving you in significant pain.

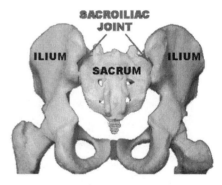

To understand creep and then material failure, take a piece of plastic. Bend it back and forth. At first, the material distorts. Then the material begins to crack, and eventually fails.

Asymmetry in the way you are built is the most common precursor to having significant back problems and the eventual disc problems as I have described as you age. From a purely mechanical perspective, without a solid base when walking, the pelvis is less stable and less able to handle loads than a symmetrical gait. Weight distribution is vitally important.

This also is why it is more likely you will throw out your back if your body is asymmetrical versus someone with a symmetrical gait or stance, which is more stable, especially when lifting things.

Typically, with overpronation, the hamstrings tighten on the side of foot flare and the person will experience tightness in the gluteal muscles (buttock) as well as the piriformis muscle; and the calf will be tight on that side. In the worse cases, the piriformis will actually turn the foot out further, causing additional painful problems in the leg and back while walking.

The body also compensates for this on the other side, tightening the quadriceps, Ileotibial band, tensor fasciae latae and adductors (structures that exist on the front and the side of your thigh), reinforcing this inappropriate way of walking.

This typically causes knee pain on the side of the tight quadriceps, meaning the kneecap will track poorly with tight adductors and quads,

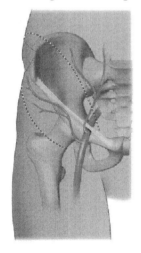 and the psoas muscle, which runs into the abdomen from the upper inner thigh, will shorten and tighten over time, further impairing appropriate movement. The oblique muscles on the same side, as well as the rectus abdominus, will tighten further torquing the hips.

As these muscles shorten, tighten, and become entrapped at the inguinal ligament (see left illustration, structure in white). It can also impair the appropriate function of nerves and blood vessels that can also become entrapped in this region, further altering the way you walk.

Eventually, your body will attempt to adjust to the asymmetry with less than desirable consequences. Typically, the mechanical firing patterns (the way muscles coordinate movement in the body) will be altered over time, reinforcing a poor functional pattern both neurologically and structurally with a tightening of the myofascia (connective tissue), setting the stage for chronic pain and inflexibility in the upper body.

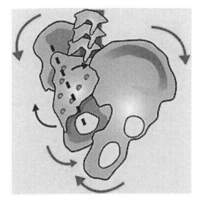

The result is a counter-rotation of the pelvis, also called tortipelvis, created when someone with an asymmetrical body style coordinates power differently in the right and left sides. In my practice, I commonly see a tightening of the lower back on one side and a tightening of the anterior hip on the other, which creates torsion at the pelvis. Most people recognize this as back pain and groin pain after standing a while or walking in the mall. If the problem is advanced, this affects their knees and hips, and the person can experience not only back pain but also joint pain throughout the legs, hips, back and upper extremities.

Think of a suspension bridge supported by wires as shown in the photograph at the right. The engineers designed the bridge so the ropes are symmetrically placed and the force is balanced on both sides keeping the roadway level and stable. Imagine what would happen if the ropes on one side contracted. The roadway would no longer be level. It would distort. The ability to hold the weight of the cars

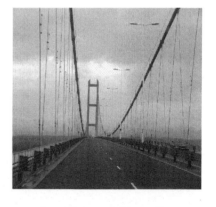

would now be compromised. The same is true then the muscles pull on the pelvis unevenly.

When pelvis torsion is well developed, these people can walk a while and then may have to sit down due to the pain in the back, neck and shoulders. They often believe they are tired, or that this is normal since they have always functioned like this. Also, over time, the muscles and ligaments will tighten more as they age as they naturally attempt to tolerate the chronic pain produced when the pelvis functionally locks up, which markedly affects how their body can move even more.

The body derives power and mechanical leverage from the pelvis. Distortion of the pelvis is responsible for many neck and shoulder problems and goes largely ignored because it may not be symptomatic other than the person saying they are inflexible. In the United States, this is a condition most successfully treated with manipulation in chiropractic offices and in some osteopathic facilities.

One More Reason to Blame Your Parents...
Genetics

Many of us remember our parents comparing who their children looked like the most. Did you get dad's nose, moms chin, dad's bald spot, etc? Unless you were adopted, your gene pool consists of the many generations that came before you in your family. Of course, adopted children face the same challenges with the complication of not being in the position to look across the room and visually see reasons for their biomechanical issues. Certain features such as the color of your skin, hair, and other body features are shared with other generations and ultimately, became part of your makeup.

Certain genes are recessive, meaning they have a one-in-four chance of appearing if both parents have the characteristics, and tending to skip generations; whereas dominant genes do not skip generations and are most likely to occur in each successive generation.

> When it comes to why your joints hurt consider that,
>
> "Genetics is a cruel hoax played on an unsuspecting public."
>
> - Dr. William Charschan

You may inherit your parents' good looks, but you may also get other less desirable features such as the tendency toward high cholesterol, high blood pressure and other potential health issues. This is true of some inherited genetic diseases that run in certain families. That is genetics, the good, bad and the ugly.

Most parents notice their infant's facial features such as the nose, or compare their own baby photo to their newborn child. When you look at your aging family members beyond the facial features, your uncles and aunts, you may notice that their shoulders are more rounded, and they become more knock-kneed. You may notice other body features. You will also notice that as you age and compare to pictures of your relatives that you resemble them not only facially but also in the way you are built because you are all from similar gene pools. In other words, you do not only have some facial features in common, but also body style, legs, feet, etc.

The point is that certain features will occur in every generation while certain features skip a generation; and body style passes collectively from generation to generation.

In other words, if your dad and mom have flat feet, chances are that you and your siblings have it, too. If your mom and dad are tall, it is likely you and your siblings are also tall. If your mom and dad are built with a significant amount of asymmetry, with one foot that flares out or turns in as compared to the other side, you likely have that trait too.

Of course, there is observationally learned behavior, too. Children learn by copying. There is well-documented proof of "mirroring". Most of us do it unconsciously. For example, if you are sitting across the table from someone and he leans forward, you tend to lean forward. He leans back. You lean back. He picks up his fork. You pick up your fork. If you have a duck-footed stance, and your shoulders roll forward, even if not genetically pre-disposed, your children could mimic you, creating otherwise mechanical and functional issues.

When children are very young, they first begin to roll over and crawl. Then they pull themselves up in an attempt to stand, and then finally try to take their first steps, modeling those around them. As children begin to walk, and grow into toddlerhood, they all walk flat-footed. Usually between the ages of three and six, their gait develops and they begin to walk more like adults, and their feet naturally begin to turn out.

Since some children progress faster than others do, parents do naturally become concerned. It had heard many stories about children wearing special shoes or other corrective devices that would ensure the feet turn out. While the intention of these devices is to change a normal adaptation, this process usually occurs on its own without the help of bracing.

By age six, you can see which child is developing asymmetry and gait related issues affecting their legs spine and upper bodies. We develop the arches in our fee (shaped by genetics). Children with gait and asymmetry related issues tend to be less flexible, with difficulty touching their toes. They tend to experience pain while they grow called "growing pains." They experience pain in their shins when they run, referred to as shin splints. They develop knee pain or Osgood Schlatters disease, which is an extreme version of shin splints that results in a bump developing at the tibial plateau (the front of the shin just below the knee) with growth spurts.

Other children adapt so their heels do not touch the floor as they walk (toe walkers). They can even have an uneven gait, where one side is tight in the back and the other tight in the front causing under-striding on the side of foot flare and over-striding on the opposite side, a common cause of back and neck pain and pulled muscles during athletic and other activities.

Addressing Genetically Caused Musculoskeletal Issues

The good news is that we can address the most common causes of back pain, leg pain, hip pain, neck pain and shoulder pain. These conditions originate in the feet, the bodies foundation. This is a condition called foot overpronation. This inherited trait causes the front of the foot to roll in excessively while you stand and walk, overly stressing the foot joints, ankle joints, knee joints and other joints in the body.

We often associate foot overpronation with flat feet that have flexible arches. The more the foot toes out, the more the knee rotates in having the effect of increasing the stress on the ankle, knee and hip and secondarily, causing a shortening and tightening of the leg muscles in the back of the involved leg.

You can also have high arches and overpronate if the foot toes out enough. If this effect is asymmetrical, with one foot toeing out more than the other foot, this causes chronic problems for this person.

Secondarily, the hip flexors (psoas is the main hip flexor and the strongest muscle in the body), the abdominal muscles, the gluteal muscles, the multifidii and the quadratus lumborum (main muscles making up your core) will tighten and alter the way the region functions in an asymmetrical fashion. The oblique and rectus abdominus muscles (stomach muscles) will then pull the shoulder forward on that side, which causes the shoulder girdle to function improperly. Typically, the entire side gets tight and, secondarily, the opposite side strains if the opposite foot turns out less. When you look at someone from the back built this way, instead of a smooth movement of the hips, you see an exaggerated movement, where one side moves and the other side does not. The more asymmetrical the gait, the more the person has a tendency to waddle from side to side.

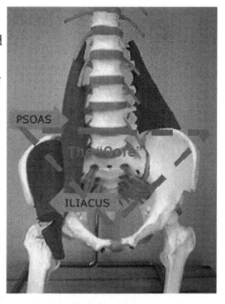

As we grow, and as these movement patterns become reinforced by a shortening and adaptation of the myofascia (the connective tissues covering muscles and other structures), the neurological system via mechanoreception(the body's ability to subconsciously know where your leg is going in relationship to movement), ligamentous adaptation and eventual muscular tightness from compensation.

An asymmetric gait overstresses the lower back joints, strains the pelvic joints, and creates pain while walking as well as problems in the shoulders and neck. In most cases, this is the source of chronic back pain, neck pain, shoulder and shoulder joint aches and pain, jaw problems, knee pain and other painful conditions.

In the worst cases, the rib cage will distort, causing chronic neck and shoulder pain and problems in the rotator cuff (shoulder joint) because of improperly functioning ribs that need to move during shoulder motion.

An asymmetric gait also causes shoulder blade pain, chronic neck stiffness and shoulder joint pain with clicking from the opposite shoulder that is strained.

Additional related conditions are carpal tunnel syndrome, elbow pain, wrist pain, and pain in the hands and thumb from poor function of the upper kinetic chain. The upper back spinal joints or thoracic segments rotate toward the side of overpronation as well, causing shoulder blade

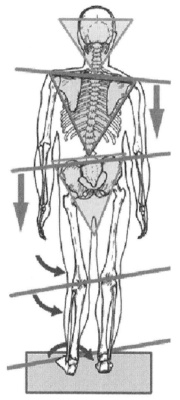

and neck pain since the neck requires proper movement of the lumbar and thoracic joints and the surrounding musculature to move freely without restriction.

Pain more often, but not always, felt on the side of strain and many people describe popping of joints when this occurs. The joints in the pelvis, lower back, upper back, neck as well as your other extremities are designed for a specific amount of motion as you walk. If you lock up one side, and the other side strains, you most often feel pain on the side of strain as you walk.

Your body develops poor movement patterns as it intuitively compensates to allow you to walk as level and efficiently as possible within the confines of your current mechanical situation body style. As you walk with these limitations for an extended period, you place strain on the joints in the pelvis and secondarily on the spinal joints above. In general, you will feel pain or a feeling of kinked or displaced joints wherever the joints are straining beyond their normal mobility.

Moreover, whenever you have hypo mobility (joints that move too little or are locked up), you tend also have joints that compensate with hyper mobility (joints moving too much).

Sufferers of chronic neck pain, headaches and shoulder pain should have their gait, body style and pelvis checked. Almost all have problems in the lower body. However, sufferers may not even realize these causes for their problems exist because if they are used to being tight and inflexible. It 'feels' normal, it may not be 'painful', or they are so accustomed to the level of pain that they do not interpret it as pain.

If we are stiff all the time, and have always been this way, we assume it is normal and just believe we are inflexible. We typically begin to develop these traits at the age of three. The way our body usually functions is our frame of reference and we consider it the norm to move and feel a certain way, since this is all we have ever known. Think of it this way, an incredibly near-sighted person who has never worn corrective prescription eyeglasses sees the world as blurry. One day, he puts on a pair of corrective glasses and recognizes all he was missing. It is only when we begin to experience pain outside our frame of reference or what we are accustomed to, we consider this abnormal.

Asymmetrical gait is typical in the sufferers of back pain, sciatic pain, and herniated disc, neck pain (especially with an acute stiff neck), knee pain (especially acute knee pain) and chronic shoulder joint pain.

From a health care practitioners point of view, having the knowledge to be able to screen all patients for gait issues first, is a huge asset, since most people with these complaints have subtle gait abnormalities as the cause, and the back symptoms occur secondarily.

As a patient, you want a health care provider who really understands the gait process, and will evaluate you, not just the presented symptoms. Your health care practitioner needs to make you aware of these other areas of involvement, instead of just relying on the areas of symptoms. You want a health care practitioner who will be thorough, look past the obvious symptoms and give you information and guidance so you can enjoy an overall better quality of life.

I use a patient's list of complaints and history as a roadmap to the problems he is currently experiencing, and can often make him aware of other symptoms that can occur in the future because those symptoms are usually part of the existing mechanical problem, rather than the problem itself.

A scientific approach based on what I have told you would never just look at the lower back if the person complained of lower back pain. A scientific practitioner would not just look at the knee when evaluating knee pain considering other parts of the body can create the condition, even if the history sounds like the cause was obvious.

A shoulder problem requires a look at the entire body. Headache treatment and prescription would not come before a complete evaluation of body style and posture because it is a vital part of understanding why the person has headaches.

A scientific approach evaluates and tests function, applies functionally restorative treatment, and is typically able to see an instantaneous change upon retesting. If not, the practitioner can quickly continue with further evaluation to understand why the response was not as intended or expected, thereby assuring a more reliable outcome.

A scientific approach will apply knowledge of function, and understand body mechanics, cause and effect, and work on cause, not effect.

You get the idea.

We need to make a habit of thinking outside the symptom-disease box and get out of the allopathic paradigm of prescribing medication without understanding first the pain and inflammatory causes and treating the musculoskeletal system as a series of discrete mishaps and diseases (disc disease, degenerative joint disease, Fibromyalgia disease).

Science does not equal drugs and rehabilitation. Science equals a thorough evaluation, and a good understanding of why things are not working well and then, coming up with solutions that resolve the malfunctions in a predictable fashion.

Body Mechanics and the Painful Conditions It Causes in way Consumers can Understand

As a rule, it is normal to avoid pain. It is evolutionarily hard-wired into us. And today, with the busy lives we lead, who wouldn't want to find the easiest solution to relieve pain so you can function and care for yourself, your children, your family, and fulfill your obligations for your employer. Unfortunately, we often ignore our own needs, and sacrifice for others.

One coping mechanism is ignoring small discomforts when we are younger, especially because they appear to go away. We are taught that sometimes things hurt, "to deal with it" and "to tough it out" until the pain goes away on its own.

The average person has no idea that his body style has much to do with a great deal of the pain or stiffness he experiences during his lifetime. As a rule, people believe the way they feel is normal. If you are always stiff and you do not know of any other reality, this is your only frame of reference and you consider this normal.

Body Style, Kinetic Chains and Firing Patterns

Body style (the way you are built) will determine how your body ultimately works. It will determine if you are destined to have joint pain or painful lower back, neck, shoulder, knee and other conditions we commonly treat in my office.

In the early 1990's, I came across a study published by a Podiatric researcher, Professor Brian Rothbart (http://www.rothbartsfoot.bravehost.com).

Professor Rothbart proposed a theory he called bio-implosion based on an engineering model of the effect of gravity on the human frame secondary to the shape of the feet. This appealed to me on two levels.

First, before choosing chiropractic, I was a mechanical engineering major in college. Secondarily, just a few short years after going into private practice I was already convinced of the importance of foot shape and position and understood the reasons with some help from my engineering background. In 1995, I knew there was more of a connection between what happened at the ground from someone's gait (the way they walked) and the information Dr. Leahy imparted to us during the early days of Active Release Techniques ®. I used what I had learned and even created my own theories trying different things on different patient's which worked with favorable results. This led me to develop many of my own theories on how things worked. Years later, Thomas Myers and his book on Anatomy Trains helped confirm my suspicions regarding how the myofascia acts on human movement depending on the forces placed upon it.

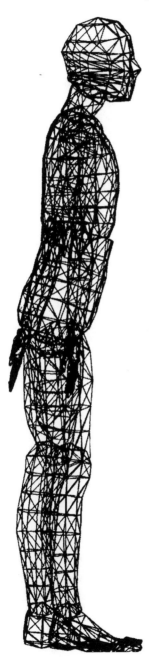

Excited by the Professor Rothbart's findings, I expanded on the information, authoring the first article of many called the Basic Pronation Accommodation Pattern published in Dynamic Chiropractic. You can find the original article and others on www.chiroweb.com in their online archive by searching the article title.

I then expanded these thoughts to include kinetic chain activity and the effect of overpronation on the kinetic chains. Kinetic chains are series of joints that affect each other. The ankle, knee and hip are a kinetic chain. The shoulder, elbow and wrist are a kinetic chain.

Rothbart's model, left, shows that foot flare causes the body to lean forward. My own practice research found this to be predictably correct. In my population of thousands of chiropractic patients, all patients experiencing pain syndromes had some level of Rothbart's model.

The one thing I did not discuss in detail in the article was the effect of asymmetry, which is what causes most of the problems we suffer from when we age in our joints and muscles. I needed to do a little more work to incorporate asymmetry into a cohesive theory and practice of diagnosis and treatment.

Once I fully understood the significance of Rothbart's model, I was able to predict which patient would eventually suffer from what problems with a very high degree of accuracy in my assertions. I found a reliable and repeatable method to diagnose and treat, and predict and prevent patient problems.

Based on body style, I was able to predict why people had certain problems and recognized that their history was a roadmap to why they were in pain. All I needed to do was ask the right questions to get a great understanding of the cause of a patient's problems.

I could then, with great certainty, perform evaluations already knowing why my patient was in pain, what the malfunction was and be able to reliably predict what I would see during the evaluation because of the predictability of the correlation of the history and their body style. I would be able to tell most patients what we were going to see and be 80-90% right based on assumptions drawn from body style alone.

It works like this: people more frequently feel pain in areas that are strained, and generally believe the strained side is tight (because it feels that way) and the tight side was not a problem (because it usually is asymptomatic). Many people make their problem worse by stretching the side of tightness. Since the strained side is distorted, they often increase the distortion and make themselves feel worse as they attempt to "work it out" on their own with stretches, Yoga and other methods.

It became apparent to me that if your history included the right questions asked by your doctor, your doctor could interpret the roadmap; make certain assumptions based on your body style, see if it made sense functionally and develop an effective thesis for resolving your problem cost effectively.

Wouldn't it be great if most health care providers could see right through the acute episode and come up with effective and reliable solutions for most patients without needing to resort to expensive testing and haphazard treatment regimens that often just do not work; and in many cases, exacerbate the problem?

I had an opportunity to teach this method of evaluation to a group of 62 doctors at Palmer Chiropractic College in the late 1990's.

At the conclusion of the training session, all the attending physicians saw the body differently. From this one lesson, many were now able see the body from a more functional basis; with a solid basis for their opinions regarding the real cause of a patients' suffering and have a better sense of how to solve their problem.

Possibly more important, however, was the improvement in doctor inter-reliability (the ability for more than one health care provider to agree on a diagnosis). Every physician understood how the body compensates for its mechanical deficiencies, and every physician accepted the need to diagnose and treat function, not just name the symptom and apply a therapy to it.

Of course, patients with stubborn problems often have other issues such has herniated discs, systemic disorders or other problems that do not allow the patient to improve reliably. Fortunately, these more severe problems are quite rare. However, most doctors (especially those that did not attend my training) have learned to evaluate these rare problems as though they are common in the population, which in the end leads to unnecessary testing and often does not lead to a fast and appropriate level of care and is expensive.

Why My Body Style Makes Me Hurt

You and I look like others in our families. We carry ourselves the same way, inherit adaptive traits such as the feet turning out or turning in or being flat. We inherit traits that can make us more likely to be thin, fat, or be big-boned.

Women typically have wide hips designed for child bearing. But wide hips can also make them more prone to pain from asymmetry than men, and more likely to experience injury and knee problems[63].

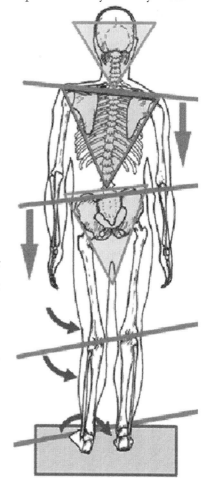

Since the body does not tolerate asymmetry well (I have come to this conclusion after many years of treating people with marked asymmetric body styles), the more asymmetrically built you are, the more mechanical problems you are likely to develop because of strain. When a body style causes one side to tighten, the other side compensates and moves, straining joints and setting up a series of events that affects the way the entire body moves. If your foot turns out on one side, the other side strains in an attempt to maintain normal movement and gait. This is why looking at a persons body style is important during any evaluation by your health care provider.

Look, again, at the model pictured left. Notice how the left foot toes out. This causes the lower leg (the shin bone also known as the tibia) to rotate in, along with the femur (thigh bone) and the knee.

This same process now stresses the hip on the same side and causes the pelvis on that same side to drop.

You can clearly see changes in how the lower back moves and how the upper back twists and rotates to accommodate these changes.

The overall effect causes the structures on the right side to experience increased stress and work inefficiently, since every joint in this series is no longer in its optimal operational position.

The body accommodates this asymmetry with muscle, connective tissue and ligamentous tightening over time on this side, and secondary changes on the opposite side as the body attempts to adjust for the increased workload.

In this example, the back of the left leg gets tighter, and the front of the right leg tightens into the hip flexors (the quads, adductors, psoas, IT band and Tensor Fasciae Latae) creating asymmetrical movement about the pelvis.

This causes you to over-stride on the right side (the leg moves too far forward when your heel strikes the ground compared to the leg on the opposite side). Meanwhile, you under-stride on the left side (your leg does not go as far as the opposite side causing you to hit the ground with your heel prematurely and increasing the force at which you hit the ground), which affects the way the joints in your pelvis move.

This torque on the pelvis ultimately translates into muscular problems above your hips, with your spine having movement that is more erratic. The deep posterior muscles along the spine (multifidii) tighten more on the side of the foot flare, the gluteal muscles tighten along with the hamstrings and you ultimately lose rotation in that hip joint causing increased stress on the hip as your foot strikes the ground.

Your leg becomes mechanically inefficient as the structure becomes tighter over time due to the accommodation of the surrounding myofascia and tissues, causing you to recruit other muscles, including the abdominal muscles, which pull the shoulder forward out of its normal working position on that side.

In the extreme, the body compensates with the entire rib cage rotating, making the mid-back joints feel locked up, causing chronic neck pain, tightness and in many people tension headaches.

Since the shoulder cannot work optimally in this position, you recruit other muscles in the region, which creates chronic painful problems in the neck, mid back and shoulder joints as well as the elbow and wrist from the lost leverage and motion in the shoulder.

Pain usually, but not always, occurs on the side of strain. In the case of the above diagram, the person is likely to experience right hip pain since this series of events will lock up the joints on the left side of the pelvis. The person will try to accommodate this in the way he/she walks. However, the motion must go somewhere.

To make up for the lack of motion on the side of foot flare, the opposite side attempts to move twice as far. Athletes who experience this in a bad way have many a pulled muscle to show for it, stress fractures or many other gait related issues. As the athlete ages, they often suffer pulled muscles frequently due to repeated strains, which are cumulative and lead to overall less flexibility. Simply, myofascia that are shortened and tightened are more likely to result in muscles that strain and fail with less provocation. This does not include probable joint damage that will occur over time as well.

These same people often experience other injuries such as shoulder blade pain or shoulder pain on the opposite side of the foot flare due to rib involvement and rib cage shift. You will read real-life case patient case studies later in the book. Meanwhile...

Since many athletes innately, and mistakenly, believe they can stretch out a tight area. The constant stretching gives them temporary relief because stretching has an anesthetic effect on tissues. Unfortunately, they are aggravating the condition by straining areas that are already strained.

While most women can experience these issues, wide-hipped women can have these problems amplified increasing the stress on the hip and knee further due to their anatomical shape.

In addition, it is not unusual for someone to believe they are experiencing a heart attack due to pain actually caused by the ribs, the surrounding muscles and their insertion points. Any emergency room doctor can tell you many people experiencing chest pain have the pain for reasons other than a heart attack, and you guessed it; pain from the tightened muscles, fascia and the effect on the rib cage. This is an expensive way to diagnose muscle spasm.

A recent patient experienced similar symptoms to those described here. She presented with rib pain, chronic hip pain and chronic neck stiffness. She learned to tolerate the pain and tightness until it stopped her from playing tennis. She could no longer hit her serve without pain, and she had to alter the way she ran for a ball due to the strain on the ribs.

Ultimately, we solved her pain and functional problems non-surgically and without prescription medication using a simple and safe combination of shoe inserts and myofascial release to loosen her core muscles and hip flexors. Importantly, during treatment, I advised her to cease her exercise regimen until her core muscle flexibility improved. She followed instructions, kept her appointments, and was hitting ace serves again in no time.

So, Let Me Ask You...

- Are you plagued by conditions diagnosed and treated using the symptom model that may have explanations and solutions as logical and simple as those discussed in this book?
- Are you starting to consider that your shoulder or knee did not "just go bad" because of an activity and that maybe you have another problem that the activity just triggered?
- Are you starting to think that maybe you do not just have a "weak back?"
- Are you beginning to believe that stuff does not "just happen", because you are getting older and that maybe your back problems,

knee problems, headaches and other issues related to musculoskeletal system have mechanical explanations with mechanical solutions?
- Are you intrigued by the idea that there is a reason for all your
  problems and a real possibility that there is a way you can improve the way you feel and function without the use of expensive
  medical tests, harmful drugs or dangerous surgeries?

Then keep reading…

The Hidden Cause of Muscular Tightness; Firing Patterns

When you see someone built asymmetrically, with foot flare dominant on one side, you are likely looking at an individual who experiences pain and tightness. The greater his body's asymmetry, the more problems he is likely to experience.

As muscles tighten around joints because of the general inefficiency in body style and mechanics, not only do the joints strain more than is normal for the joint to tolerate, but so do the muscles, connective tissues and tendons surrounding that joint. They will shorten and tighten due to repeated micro tears and injuries.

Dr. Michael Leahy of Active Release Technique® fame, talked about the Cumulative Injury Cycle. He described what happens to people who develop cumulative trauma such as carpal tunnel syndrome and other repetitive strain type conditions.

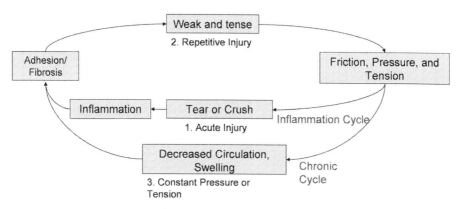

"Printed with permission of Dr. Michael Leahy, Active Release Techniques LLC."

He theorized that a loss of oxygen to the tissues causes tightening of the tissues and as the tissues tighten, it increases the strain on the tissues, which causes them to get even tighter. This causes the tissues to fibrose (become fibrous and tough) and creates chronic pain and tightness as the tissues continue to lose oxygen and are forced to work in an oxygen-deprived state. See his chart on his theory extrapolated from the current literature.

His model, although geared to explaining cell compromise due to compression in the tissues, partly explains why muscles and the surrounding fascia tighten in response to repeated loads. We can also use his model to explain why people with body style issues will, over time, compensate and tighten in response to flat feet, foot flare and overall body asymmetry.

Another piece of the equation concerns firing patterns. Firing patterns are the orders of action the different muscles follow in order to move a joint properly.

When muscles are weakened and tightened from processes such as the cumulative injury cycle, they have less power and less leverage and, therefore, impaired coordination when used during normal activities.

If the body cannot move a joint properly, it recruits other muscles to help; meaning the body uses muscles not designed for the task to compensate. Muscles that fire poorly cause other areas to tighten up because these areas are performing tasks for which they are not designed. The result of chronic recruitment with poor movement coordination is chronic pain and tightness in the muscles that are recruited in to help with the impaired movement. Over time, the body adapts neurologically and "naturally" supports this impaired method of motion as if it is the norm.

A common example of this is shoulder blade pain.

When a shoulder is firing poorly, the person is likely to experience wrist, elbow and hand pain as well as numbness from compensation as the shoulder loses flexibility and strength. A poorly functioning shoulder is unstable and has a compromised mechanical advantage. To demonstrate, when I ask a patient with shoulder pain to push their hand against mine, he finds it difficult and experiences pain in the shoulder that was the main complaint.

When this is the case, and I place the persons opposite side hand on the shoulder blade of the side I tested, he feels those muscles tightening when they should not be.

This phenomenon is the person recruiting their upper and middle traps and neck muscles as they attempt to resist my arm. When I change the angle of pull by pushing their shoulder backward (see Example 1), the patient usually immediately feels they can push against me with more force and notices the shoulder blade tightens less.

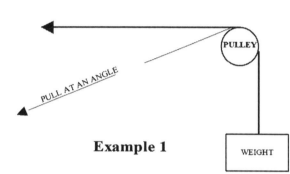

Example 1

This pulley analogy explains from an engineering standpoint the concept of leverage and how the angle of pull can make a structure either more or less mechanically efficient.

Unless a person is trying to push something, pull something, or lift something heavy, he is not aware of whether he has leverage or not. He is aware of being tight, or being in pain.

If you have a poorly functioning shoulder, your neck, upper shoulder and shoulder blade muscles typically recruit and tighten as they help compensate for a poorly coordinating joint.

Recruitment is often the reason for chronic pain in many areas of the body. Even simple things such as turning the wheel in your car can cause recruitment into the shoulder, neck and blade if the shoulder is not working properly.

People suffering chronic pain and immobility need not feel like their only choice is to experience tightness all the time. This is why the diagnosis of poor firing patterns is critical. Once corrected, many chronic pains or tightness and stiffness conditions significantly improve or resolve altogether.

The knowledge and technology exists to help people who are either stiff or in pain all the time. We need to teach physical therapists, chiropractors and other manual treatment providers to properly recognize, diagnose and treat these types of problems. Primary care providers should learn about how this works as well and refer these patients to health care providers who are proficient at evaluating and treating these problems for long-term relief without medication and without surgery.

Unfortunately, the current health care system does not teach doctors much about how the body works mechanically as whole, as it does to evaluate a painful area, name it, place a diagnostic code on it, and then direct treatment to it based on the diagnostic code. Most of your health care providers may never really understand why you are in pain and what causes it because they are evaluating and treating the symptom, rather than the problem.

Patients often bring me theories as to why they hurt, wanting a professional opinion as to why they are in pain. By understanding the underlying mechanisms described here, I can easily demonstrate to the person why the area hurts and, combined with his history, develop working theories about why he is in pain and treatment solutions that are helpful in resolving his condition.

Understanding how joints interact with each other allows your health care practitioner to show someone how their body works and understand why they continue to tighten up and find themselves in pain.

The Truth about Pain in the Lower Leg, Women and Childbirth

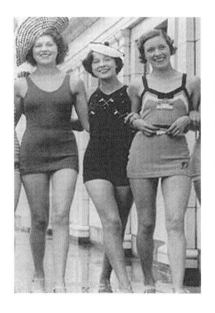

The way your foot makes contact with the ground determines whether it functions well, or functions poorly. Even with a healthy arch, if your foot toes out too much, your knee and hip rolls in more than your body can tolerate, creating a cascade of events of inappropriate motion throughout the hips, spine, ribs, shoulders, neck ankles and feet, as well as the elbows and wrists.

A woman is likely affected by this more than a male because of a wider pelvis which increases the angle that the femur attaches to the tibia, which, in turn, increases the strain at the knee and kneecap, making you more prone to knee injuries[64].

Since foot overpronation, foot flare and body asymmetry is inherited, typically a woman who inherits the same foot problem as her dad or her brother can experience symptoms that are worse than her male counterpart, especially since her hips are wider.

For the same reason, it is also no coincidence that many women experience increased lower back pain after pregnancy. Not only is a new mother constantly lifting her newborn, but also it is natural for a woman's hips to spread somewhat before and during childbirth from the stretching of the ligaments in the pelvis as her body prepares for the birth, and then as the child physically passes through the pelvis[65].

Since these traits existed prior to the pregnancy and the birth of the baby, the change in width further increases the angle at which her knee works(known medically as the Q Angle -http://en.wikipedia.org/wiki/Q_angle#Q_angle), negatively affecting kneecap efficiency and further straining the joints in the lower kinetic chain[66].

If the woman has an asymmetrical build, she is even more likely to experience pain in her knees and back as one side becomes tight, causing the opposite side to strain in the pelvis and secondarily affecting her upper body movement. Childbirth is a miraculous event. It also increases the load on the knees and exacerbates any functional problems that existed prior to the pregnancy, which may have been asymptomatic.

Another problem a woman experiences from childbirth is coccyx related back pain. Some believe the coccyx to be a vestigial remnant of a human tail eliminated through evolution. Regardless, during childbirth, the pressure of the baby displaces the mother's coccyx as it progresses through the birth canal. A woman with wider hips is more likely to have problems in this area because the wider hips more easily expose the coccyx to trauma, such as falls and other impacts[67].

Pain can radiate down the leg, often aggravated by sitting. Many women suffering from this have tolerated it for a while, often getting frustrated when treatment methods that should work do not work. Here is why...

When treating the coccyx, it is not enough to manipulate only the structure because the musculature and ligaments are often too tight. I have personally treated hundreds of women with this condition by first loosening up the surrounding musculature and then using tension on the surrounding tissues to gently place the coccyx in motion. Even if the coccyx was fractured years ago, patients tend to respond well to manipulation.

There are cases when a coccyx may be pushed too far in and require gynecological assistance with internal manipulation; however, in my experience this is rarely necessary.

Flat Feet, Foot Flare, Short First Toes, Aching Ankles and More

When a flat or low arch combined with toeing out exists, you have set the stage for all sorts of probable future pains and problems. For example, knee pain, foot pain, plantar fasciitis, shin pain, Achilles tendon problems, calf pain and other problems extending up the lower kinetic chain; the series of joints that affect each other such as the ankle, knee and hip that comprise the lower kinetic chain.

The problem is amplified when a person has a short first toe, which decreases the mechanical advantage in the foot as it hits the ground and increases stress on the second and third toes when walking. A short first toe has been known to cause other mechanical overuse problems in the foot including Morton's neuroma'.

As described by Mayoclinic.com, Morton's neuroma involves a thickening of the tissue around one of the nerves leading to your toes. In some cases, Morton's neuroma causes a sharp, burning pain in the ball of your foot. Your toes may also sting, burn or feel numb.

When someone has foot flare on one side and the other side either turns out

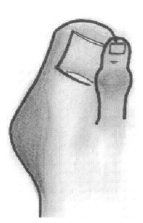

less or supinates (turns in, often associated with a high stiff arch), the changes at the pelvis tighten the posterior leg on the side of foot flare from compensation. The other side will tighten in the front of the thigh, the lateral leg and deep hip flexors on that side. The long-term result of this asymmetry is a pattern of tightness in the myofascia (connective tissue that surrounds the muscles) surrounding the person's core muscles (the muscles surrounding a person's mid-section). The effect will torque the pelvis creating a loss of leverage which will secondarily make the legs and upper back tight as they compensate to work around a poorly functioning core..

The same thing happens as a bunion develops because it, too, causes you to lose the mechanical advantage in the foot as you walk because the toe is no longer straight, causing your foot to roll in.

Bunions are prevalent with people whose feet turn out because foot flare causes increased lateral stress on the toe. Over time, it migrates laterally; causing the joint to change in character and often becomes painful. The other problem is that as the bunion progresses, your gait changes and the foot tends to roll in more creating problems in other parts of the foot, ankle and kinetic chain. People with bunions try to accommodate to the condition by wearing wider shoes, which generally do not fit as well as shoes sized correctly, and can cause a series of other issues.

The Problem with Help These Days

Over time, the myofascia accommodates to the forces involved resulting in the way we hold ourselves at rest while we sit, stand and even lay down. Many published methods rely on stretching and other techniques, like the Alexander Technique used to teach a person how to sit or stand properly. Some methods, such as the Feldenkrais Method, theorize that movement patterns are learned and must be re-taught.

Thomas Myers in his previously mentioned book about Anatomy Trains has shown the myofasia exists in tracts that affect how we move and that the old ideas of how muscles work individually are untrue and do not represent how the body actually functions mechanically. Myers' research is turning our current educational knowledge of muscle function on its head.

While attempting to help a patient reach the ideal position and teaching alternative movement is admirable and necessary, the problem is that posture during standing or sitting is a reflection of how our muscular system has adapted to our structure, and what that adaptation does when we attempt to level ourselves against gravity while standing, sitting or even laying down. These methods and techniques are trying to work around the problem instead of fixing the problem.

Although these schools of thought are part of the process of changing how the body can work, you must undo the changes that have occurred

Resource Box

You can find Dr. Thomas Myers' books and material at:

www.anatomytrains.com

You can find Dr. Moshe Feldenkrais' books and material at:

www.achievingexcellence.com

For more about the Alexander Technique pioneered by Australian actor F. M. Alexander to relieve excess muscle tension visit:

www.alexandertechnique.com

in the fascial system and then reeducate the area. Attempting to retrain muscles that are very tight without taking into account structure or work toward more normal movement patterns while restoring the ability to perform these movements without myofascial treatment is a lesson in futility.

The bottom line is that your body develops its structure based on genetic predisposition. Your body adapts to this structure. If the structure is asymmetrical, over time your body tightens in response to the side with foot flare and strains on the opposite side, causing the connective tissue (the myofascia) to get tighter over time, literally cementing these movements in place as your body neurologically adapts to moving in this restricted fashion and convincing itself this is normal behavior.

These accommodations affect the way you walk because one leg will under-stride. The back of your leg gets tight due to tightness in the buttock, with secondary tightening of the hamstring muscle behind the thigh, and then a tightening of the calf on the same side.

This eventually affects the deep muscles against the spine, including the multifidii and the erector spinae. The side opposite the tight side accommodates this and over strides. The back of the opposite leg is looser, but the front is tight, resulting in excessive forces in the hip joints, knee joints, sacroiliac joints and other secondary stresses affecting the spine, rib cage and shoulders joints, elbows and even the wrists. This is a common cause for chronic back pain and sciatic-like symptoms as well as pelvic torsion.

The Harmful Effect of Overpronation and Loss of Leverage

Overpronation causes inefficient angles for the muscles in the lower leg to work. The effect is torsion of the pelvis from which we derive leverage when walk, run and perform our normal activities.

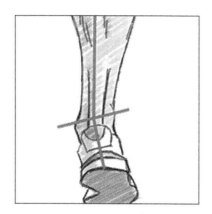

Overpronation causes the tibia to rotate in too much as the foot flares out resulting in many knee pain syndromes. Problems include kneecap mistracking and grinding, chondromalacia (a breakdown of the cartridge under the kneecap or in the knee), tendonosis of the hamstring (chronic scarring inside the tendon creating pain) and gastroc muscular insertions, meniscus tears, cruciate ligament tears as well as long term damage to other structures that surround and accommodate to inappropriate knee mechanics.

Since the torqued pelvis loses a mechanical advantage as it distorts, the firing patterns (the way muscles coordinate to efficiently move the body) change causing an increased workload on the legs, hips, back muscles and abdominal musculature. Over time, improper loads and inefficient movement causes significant tightening of the legs, hips, core muscles, upper back, neck and arms. The entire body is negatively affected.

Typically, a person with this issue may experience pain called shin splints in his legs when walking or running. This is

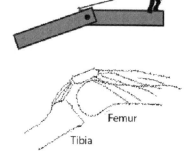

Femur

Tibia

the result of the muscles in the front of his shins becoming tight and pulling against their bony insertions.

His knees may crack as he crouches down because with extreme knee bending this type of posture causes the kneecap to rotate, and in the worst cases, slip to the side. As the hip muscles tighten on the side of overpronation, the effect is the calf tightens in the back of the leg.

Many patients I see seek evaluation and treatment for significant knee pain. They are always more than a little surprised to learn that their problem is a back and foot problem, causing the muscles to tighten into the back of the knee. This is because the knee is a conduit through which forces pass, with the kneecap acting as a pulley. If the pulley works poorly, the person eventually develops symptoms in the knee. Tight quadriceps due to poor pelvic and core stability causes excess tightness at the kneecap and it becomes a poor pulley system.

Because these forces come from the ground and pelvis stability, it is essential that we address problems from the ground up with appropriate footwear or orthotics and balance out the muscles in the pelvis and the muscles surrounding the knee with methods such as myofascial release, strengthening them to reduce the forces at the knee. This flies in the face of conventional medical wisdom, which labels the condition, diagnoses and treats only the area of pain, which in this case is the knee.

Unfortunately, the most doctors send patients with knee pain for therapy directed at the knee with the belief that the quadriceps and other surrounding musculature are weak and need strengthening. The big problem with this approach is that the weakness is due to tightening of the musculature and structures surrounding the knee because of compensation. Attempting to load up the leg with "therapeutic" exercises without understanding how or why it became tight and weak is a bad diagnosis followed by an ineffective treatment that has a good chance to make the problem worse.

Of course, it is just as bad ignoring or leaving the problem unaddressed. The net effect of which is pain.

Runners and both amateur and professional athletes can experience stress fractures in either the foot or the tibia because of compensation during the constant usage. I have seen patients for these issues who have told me they had stress fractures with care rendered only at the symptomatic region. By not correcting the underlying structure that created the problem, over time patients experience more stress fractures and many other painful problems[68.]

The connective tissues surrounding the ankle also tightens over time when overpronation and foot flare is present, as well as the Achilles tendon losing flexibility from the tightening of the hamstring and calf and the constant pounding during the gait cycle.

Typically, people with moderate to severe foot overpronation and foot flare are heavy heel strikers with very tight hamstrings, gluteal muscles, and calves. Typically, adhesions form in the myofascia on the posterior part of the knee, adversely affecting the calf muscles. The effect causes Achilles Tendonosis since the forces cause micro tears in the tendon that lose flexibility over time.

People who tear the Achilles tendon often do so because of this loss of flexibility. A tight structure is primed to tear when the right force is applied to it. The calf acts as a shock absorber, of sorts. A chronically tight calf due to body style issues makes a poor shock absorber. The bottom of the foot tightens (the plantar fascia), the joints in the foot and ankle move less (and in the worst cases actually jam) creating chronic foot pain, stress to the twenty-six different bones in the foot, the heel and the ankle, and, eventually, results in inappropriate knee motion.

It is also common for someone with very tight heel chords to be unable to tolerate a shoe insert such as a foot orthotic because the effect is a tightening of the plantar fascia (connective tissue on the bottom of the foot) and soreness in the tissues from the chronic stress. When the person places the insert designed to raise the arch and prevent him from turning out his foot, the bottom of the foot becomes uncomfortable with the arch in place because the foot is unable to sit on top of the insert due to plantar fascial stiffness.

To correct this problem, first, the health care provider should check the device to see that it was made and fitted correctly. Then, the health care provider should loosen the calf, back of the knee and plantar fascia, which would improve the patient's gait mechanics and creating symmetry that will help prevent the patient from slamming his foot into the ground.

Lower Back Pain, Sciatica and Lower Back Disc Syndromes

Why Lumbar **Discs Go Bad.**

Many people with lower back pain have had an MRI ordered as a diagnostic tool. However, as confirmed by various studies, many people have defects in the discs in their back and yet display no symptoms [69, 70, 71]. Therefore, an MRI can show a defect, but not necessarily the underlying cause of a patient's back pain. That is why I tell patients to allow a short trial of care before we do a powerful imaging study. Since most people improve during the trial of chiropractic care, we avoid many unnecessary referrals, and greatly improve the cost effectiveness of treatment. We can eliminate many imaging studies by allowing an adequate trial of an effective intervention.

A problem that is unresponsive to a two-to-three week trial of care is more severe and can require a different type of care or necessitate a referral to a different type of specialist. If your lower back does not improve with a course of treatment, then the MRI or CAT scan is an appropriate further evaluation to determine intensity or appropriateness of the current care plan. This, however, is just a small percentage of the population. Why screen everyone if only a small percentage of people require a referral. It clearly makes better sense to evaluate, treat, look for response and then test if necessary.

It is true that you cannot accurately diagnose a disc herniation without an MRI or a CAT scan evaluation. Again, the problem is that the true mechanical cause of the herniation is not investigated. How did the herniation occur? Why does it exist?

It is so important to look beyond the obvious. If a person's body mechanics predisposes them to having problems in the discs of their back, how much are doctors really helping the patient by obsessing on the disc problem shown on the test and ignoring the gait-related issue that created it? The answer is that it is usually related to gait (the way we walk).

To understand this concept fully, you must understand that any naturally occurring asymmetry in the feet is eventually affecting the lower back. When one foot flares out, the hip drops with each step. The stress

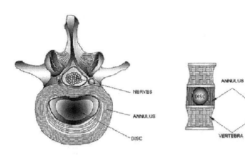

within the fibers of the disc increases noticeably because as the hip has exaggerated movement, so do the motion segments, or vertebrae, in your back.

The lumbar disc consists of a jelly-like material on the inside, with a fibrous outside. As shown in the diagram, the inside of a healthy disc is round enough to allow the joint on top to move about freely in many directions.

The outer material, called the annulus, is fibrous and tough. The discs in the lumbar spine are designed to allow a significant amount of movement between each segment, limited by the facet joints (the joints in the back of each vertebra that connect each segment together in the back adding stability to the joint).

The Lumbar facet joints and discs are relatively unprotected from excessive loads, unlike the thoracic spine (mid back) which has ribs to better stabilize the region.

If the motion in the pelvis is inappropriate or markedly restricted due to asymmetry, a significant amount of additional strain transfers to the lumbar facet joints and discs.

This is why symmetry in your body is critical. Symmetry allows for equally distributed forces through the pelvis and the rest of the spine. It also provides better mechanical advantage allowing muscles to coordinate movement resulting in better overall function.

A lack of symmetry causes one side of the pelvis to tighten (hypo mobility), and the other side to move too much (hyper mobility). These excessive forces transfer to the motion segments in the lumbar spine, including the discs, which then move excessively. The typical result is back pain and many painful spinal problems.

This excessive movement can eventually cause the *outer* fibers in the disc to fail, not unlike a piece of plastic that you continually bend until it fails. Engineers know this process as creep, described in detail earlier in the book.

Eventually, the stress causes fibers *within* the disc to fail. When they do, the person can experience a considerable amount of pain due to pain fibers in the disc[72]. On an MRI, damage to internal fibers within the disc is seen as a disc bulge. A bulge can indicate that fibers in the disc have been disrupted and the internal material may have lost is shape, which alters the way the joint works[73].

The literature suggests that the problem with lower back pain is much broader than what we teach doctors and most rehabilitation professionals are trained to look at. In other words, if you train people to see a problem in a limited fashion, they see it through the vision and excellence of the system that produced them. That is a very narrow viewpoint.

The reason back pain treatment is so expensive and unpredictable is that we teach methods that do not give the provider the ability to understand why back pain occurs. We introduce bits and pieces of concepts and orthopedic tests and ask physicians and therapists to put it all together by treating conditions without understanding why the condition exists. We then test the physicians and therapists based on what we taught them.

A provider who has passed his boards shows proficiency on what he was taught. Unfortunately, this leaves him at a major diagnostic disadvantage. We teach him little about body styles, patterns of function, kinetic chains and other parts of the puzzle. We do not put the pieces of the puzzle together for him in a logical and cohesive way so he can understand the mechanisms at work that cause pain.

He instead, is taught to look at the site of pain, not necessarily the mechanical cause of the problem.

Since we teach him to diagnose and treat back pain as a disease process, he treats the back pain as a disease because, based on what he was taught, he believes this is the way to effectively treat the condition. To the back pain sufferer's detriment, we gave him the passing grade that gives him the confidence that he is taking the appropriate approach.

Take, for example, a woman who had her daughter visit our office, only to become a patient herself. The daughter told our staff that her mother was likely to schedule an appointment as a new patient. At the time, however, she was sitting in her car with pain shooting down her leg.

The mother had visited her primary care physician who ordered an MRI. She was waiting for the results of her MRI evaluation before scheduling her appointment convinced that once the MRI told her why she had the pain, she could visit us for care. (Remember, MRIs only show or confirm where there is an abnormality, which may be the cause for the pain and are only part of the data needed to make a diagnostic decision.)

I asked her daughter if she had problems with her back before. She told me her mother had back issues for years. Further, per the daughter's description, a limited evaluation was performed and no treatment plan was ever put forth. She was simply taking drugs, and waiting for a referral to a surgical specialist. (Remember, two-thirds of patients are prescribed medication when they visit their physician.)

This is unconscionable and unnecessary.

In my world, we would have evaluated, possibly taken plain films, already had an idea of the underlying mechanical cause and would have placed her on a trial of care that would have up to an eighty percent chance of getting her feeling better. Eliminating the need for the MRI, which in many instances can cost more than the entire treatment of the condition, is more cost effective and appropriate.

In other words, the mother would clearly have benefited from a full history and evaluation, uncovering the chronic back pain, then treatment first, followed by high tech testing, if ever necessary.

There are those, physicians and lay-people alike, who covet the disease model, concerned about missing something important before ever touching the person. Given the case study you just read, that probably sounds ridiculous. After all, the mother went to her doctor to talk about the pain in her leg, not her back. Of course, the problem was in her back. The MRI came back showing a herniated disc. The real question her physician would not be able to answer was; "Why did my disc herniate?" Nor would her doctor be prepared to correct the problem. He would just eliminate the pain with medication refer her for injections, offer her some rehabilitation to the painful region and then refer her to a surgeon if no relief was found.

A good functional evaluation would yield an improved course of treatment for most people, and more often than not, eliminate the need for both an MRI and waiting for results, which rarely improves the functional basis for why someone is in pain.

A word to the wise physician and the concerned patient with musculoskeletal pain: evaluate functionally, treat first, test later, unless something does not seem right during the evaluation. It is highly unlikely that at good functional evaluation would not yield enough information to allow for a two -three week safe trial of care.

If you understand how the body works, you will know how to find the right practitioner for you. One who can work on solutions to the cause of your pain, rather than treat the pain symptom.

Shoulder Pain, Impingement Syndromes and the Rotator Cuff

The Shoulder Girdle

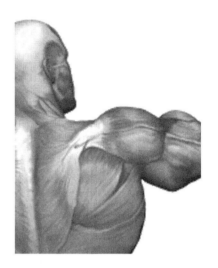

One of the most misunderstood areas of the body with regards to function is the shoulder girdle. Four muscles comprise the shoulder joint or rotator cuff: the supraspinatus, infraspinatus, teres minor and subscapularis. Many conditions of the shoulder joint cause concern due to pain and disability. These can include tears of the muscles or glenoid labrum (supportive tissue around the shoulder joint), tendon pain, muscle pain, pain with activities, stiffness and the one that is the most difficult to deal with, adhesive capsulitis (frozen shoulder).

The shoulder is directly affected by the stability of the lower body and pelvis. When you visit a doctor for your shoulder pain, he looks at the painful shoulder, performs some orthopedic tests, takes a history, diagnoses the problem and applies treatment to the region, if applicable. He may even refer you to an orthopedic surgeon since most primary care doctors are trained to send out these types of problems to specialists (usually orthopedic surgeons).

Many shoulder pain sufferers experience injections, physical rehabilitation, anti-inflammatory and muscle relaxation medications which are supposed to work on the problem. .

Typically, after an advanced imaging study such as MRI or CAT scan confirms an operable pathology as a final option when these methods fail to produce a desirable result, surgery is recommended, with no guarantee of success. Surgery, which of course has more risk than conservative, non-surgical approaches, can have variable results.

While there are some conditions that may require surgery, such as a glenoid labrum tear, full thickness tear, bony impingement, and AC joint separation, many people undergo surgery in the absence of clearly better options.

An enlightened health care practitioner looks beyond the obvious. If someone told me that the problem began while skiing and the shoulder was forced backward by a collision, the cause of the injury would seem obvious to both you and your health care provider. Obviously, the trauma caused the problem, if you never had problems with the joint before.

A while ago, a relative injured her shoulder, which required casting due to a fracture. After the cast was removed, she worked with a therapist who stretched, moved, heated, ultra sounded and performed many therapy regimens.

A year and half later, much of the pain was gone but she continued to have significant shoulder restriction on the healed side. At a family event, a bit shyly, but clearly in discomfort, she asked me to look at it briefly. The first thing I noticed was the tightness of her core muscles and the distortion of her pelvis. I loosened the tight muscles while she was standing and she was immediately able to raise the shoulder much more than before.

How could her therapist totally ignore the rest of her body?

What if, however, the shoulder was already tight and dysfunctional with no "obvious" symptoms because you were accustomed to the tightness and did not mention the tightness when you gave your history because you considered it to be normal?

If your health care practitioner ignores probing further because it was "obvious" what "caused" the injury (the trauma), your rehabilitation can be adversely affected and weeks of rehab can become months without a satisfying outcome. It is also likely that other health care providers including your therapist would miss the tightness as well.

It is outrageous that shoulder fracture rehabilitation takes one and half years without moving the case along sufficiently. In all my years of practice, I have never had a shoulder rehabilitation take that long, and that includes some very bad frozen shoulder cases.

Additionally, in this day of insurance carriers questioning every medical treatment, the case should have either been limited by the insurance carrier or capped for visits allowed for the condition. This was an across-the-board health care system failure. The best health care practitioners always question why a patient fails to progress and looks at other possibilities.

As you will recall, distortion and asymmetry in the lower body will pull the shoulders forward. A lower body evaluation should be part of every upper body evaluation, especially concerning the shoulder girdle, elbow, arm and hand, which comprises the upper kinetic chain.

Postural and body style assessment is important not only because of body style and compensation but because a person with chronic lower body involvement will eventually have his rib cage pulled forward and rotated. If this happens, one shoulder can be quite painful and appear dysfunctional due to pain avoidance apprehension. Yet, the side that is mechanically deficient may not have any symptom at all. This is because if the rib cage shifts, the opposite side becomes strained and feels kinked up or cramped and can even pop continuously with movement in both the shoulder region and even in the ribs.

You cannot find this out only by looking only at the painful area, which is what most health care providers learn in school. Health care providers are taught to evaluate the complaint using orthopedic tests, MRI and other procedures. However, they are not taught to understand body styles, compensation, firing patterns and its potential ramifications.

When evaluating your shoulder, your health care provider must evaluate the entire body, including the apparently healthy perfectly good shoulder. It is quite common, when tested, for the supposedly bad or painful shoulder to be actually functioning well mechanically and for the seemingly good shoulder to be the problem side, showing weakness and recruiting in the surrounding musculature because of a stability problem.

An enlightened practitioner evaluates everything mentioned in the previous chapters and takes a very probing, thorough history. Symptoms must be part of the history, but a thorough practitioner asks about everything after looking at your body style. The questions help uncover body style and asymmetry related problems, which is what most shoulder problems actually are.

Numbness and Pain Resulting From Postural Related Malfunction

An enlightened practitioner will know that often numbness in the hands comes from nerve entrapment inside the muscles of the shoulder joint, forearms, elbows or possibly from rib cage rotation. Unfortunately, many health care providers incorrectly assume the problem is purely neurological, coming directly from spinal nerves and their direct pathways and rely on tests such as electromyography (EMG) nerve velocity conduction (NCV) to show nerve involvement in muscle movement. Too many people have surgery for carpal tunnel syndrome as a direct result of these tests justifying the surgeries without ever being referred for a more thorough evaluation of the kinetic chain systems.

An enlightened practitioner knows how to rule out other things of consequence; like tears in the joint connective tissue, discs or bony impingement on a nerve root and then look deeper for clues as to the cause of the injury. An enlightened practitioner knows to look for nerves entrapped by the muscles and ligaments along the kinetic chains, a major source of numbness in the hands and arms, which are often mistaken for carpal tunnel syndrome.

If the patient has a tear of the supraspinatus muscle (a muscle that commonly gets impinged and damaged in the shoulder joint with chronic poor posture) on the top of the scapular spine (top of the shoulder blade), the practitioner should be able to evaluate and understand the poor mechanics that ultimately led to the painful condition.

A truly thorough practitioner will then proceed to take care of not just a lesion in the shoulder, if found, but also the mechanical cause that created it wherever it exists in the body. The mechanism of the painful joint often exists in other parts of the body, especially where the shoulder is concerned.

If your health care provider does not understand this concept, and he was taught to evaluate only the area of pain, which is what most people have learned to expect from many classes of health care providers, then you are likely to get the community standard diagnosis and treatment of the painful part. That community standard treatment will probably lead to chronic pain, pain avoidance behaviors and overall frustration because the painful part fails to respond to care.

The human body is an amazing machine with a remarkable ability to accommodate to a poor functional mechanical pattern., The result however is usually chronic pain or soreness that is perceived as normal as you become used to living with it. The problem continues to become more chronic and more limiting as you age. Since a dysfunctional kinetic chain is often the root cause of much of the chronic joint pain and back pain most people experience, other parts of the body- typically the knees, hips, and lower back can fail over time.

It is vitally important that your health care practitioner look at everything and ask many (and the right kind of) leading questions so he can rule out postural related pain issues.

Patient Care Alert:

Better diagnosis = Better treatment

This is especially important when people are considering or recovering from surgeries either directed at the shoulder or its affiliated joints. I have practical clinical evidence that many surgeries and MRI evaluations may be prevented by more thoroughness and willingness of the health care provider to look outside his symptom-disease training. As a rule, if your health care provider cannot explain why an area has impinged or calcified in the region after evaluating you, he likely has not looked at the mechanism but has instead only looked at the painful part. This type of shortsighted analysis subjects too many people to medical procedures and rehabilitation regimens that cannot possibly work.

Treating A Chronically Dysfunctional Acute Shoulder

It never makes sense to treat a pain as if it is the problem. Treating function is of ultimate importance when working with the shoulder, a dynamic joint.

If you are like most people, you take for granted activities such as walking, driving, writing, bending down to pick up things, and turning doorknobs. Like most people, you are probably unaware that the shoulder and core muscles are chiefly responsible for many of these activities occurring successfully.

The power to perform these activities comes from the shoulder working and acting appropriately, as well as from a stable core, or mid-section.

Over time, a lack of appropriate force exerted by the shoulder with core muscle imbalance causes recruitment into the forearm, wrist, palm, and neck regions (inappropriate use of other muscles to complete an action). This explains why people with dysfunctional shoulder joints develop neck pain, shoulder pain, arm pain and numbness, rib dysfunction issues, carpal tunnel syndrome and many other hand and wrist pain syndromes highlighting why it is important to evaluate the entire body, rather than just the painful part.

Recruitment tightens these muscles, negatively affects the movement at the shoulder, elbow, wrist and fingers and, over time, creates nerve entrapments that can occur anywhere along their path, which is the most common reason for numbness and pain in the arm and hand.

As much as I prefer to avoid recommending a path of medication and injection, if the area is too painful to move, it can be appropriate to receive an injection for temporary relief. Too many people, however, receive cortisone injections without appropriate care of any sort as a follow-up resulting in more severe problems in the future.

Asking a patient after the injection, "How does it feel?" and to say, "Call if it does not feel better in a couple of days," is your doctor pushing you through the door as quickly as possible. You are left wishing and hoping for a resolution while, in fact, allowing a chronic functional problem to worsen over time and present itself as other symptoms in the body.

Once the true mechanism of the shoulder pain is evaluated, your practitioner should seek to improve muscular coordination in the region (firing patterns) with the goal of improving the way your shoulder can handle gravity and daily activities. He should work toward improving your range of motion, and strengthen and loosen the other areas of the body that place tension on the shoulder as it attempts normal activities.

Treatment can initially include ice and ice massage (ice applied directly to a region) to the painful part for pain relief, but therapeutic care must also address the areas that are preventing the shoulder from working properly. These areas, as previously discussed, likely include the core muscles, leg muscles and the feet, as well as any rib cage mechanical problems that exist.

By process of elimination, an enlightened practitioner usually works by hand or with tools using myofascial release, Graston® or other techniques that address the shortened muscles and tendon fibers in the affected regions. A knowledgeable practitioner also looks for sites of nerve entrapment that can often be released by hand without resorting to expensive tests and surgeries that attack the site of the symptoms and the assumed lesion leaving the cause of the problem unchanged.

As these shortened muscles and tendon fibers in the affected regions relax, an enlightened practitioner can retest the shoulder using active evaluation techniques. Together, you and the practitioner will see an improved level of function, strength and reduction of muscular recruitment. You will notice that when the problem area is treated correctly and the practitioner tests the area again by loading it up with resistance that the painful area will either not hurt as badly or possibly not hurt at all.

This is a positive causative factor test since it proves a direct positive response to the current therapeutic intervention. This type of methodology shows instant responses, allowing a very objective path of treat, test, treat, test until a significant improvement of overall function is achieved during an office visit.

Treatment of this nature has highly predictable outcomes so there is little time wasted with therapies that do not work. By process of elimination, if a treatment is not yielding improvement during that visit, the practitioner immediately rules out the different possibilities and treats the areas of involvement until the desired outcome is achieved by the area being retested and the patient exhibits less pain and greater mechanical coordination.

The patient is re-evaluated functionally on their follow up visit to see if the area maintained the gains from the previous visit. Of course, during follow-up, questions of general well-being and progress is recorded, carefully tracking what muscles, joints and other areas that were previously treated to judge if functional expectations are met. Once a significant improvement in stability and function is reached the patient receiving treatment is ready for exercises to further improve the way the area functions.

In our office, it is not unusual to work first on the hip flexors and then test the shoulder. The reason is that if the hip flexors are causing the malfunction, or any other part including the abdominal muscles are negatively affecting shoulder function, the net effect will be an improvement of strength, a decrease of muscular recruitment and, in many cases, a decrease in symptoms, often without direct treatment toward the symptomatic part.

Significantly, this helps the patient understand that painful parts are not necessarily the problem areas.

Education is vitally important for the patient to understand how his body functions and what the pain he is experiencing really means. This knowledge makes the patient more self sufficient and able to make better choices when he experiences pain he cannot possibly manage on his own. Using treatment as an education tool illustrates to the patient that by improving hip flexors and the core, we improve the mechanics of the area that is in pain or in discomfort.

A typical and successful treatment uses the process of elimination with the most obvious and common problems addressed first and then retesting the region to see if it is not only less painful but also if it can handle an increased load appropriately.

For instance, I muscle test not only typical motions that a patient uses daily, but also individual muscles that can contribute to the overall condition. As the patient is able to tolerate more stress on the area during the treat, test, treat, test cycle, I get a reliable level of much higher function. Furthermore, the person treated usually acknowledges less pain while performing the same activity, being able to exert more force in an action that was formerly painful.

For example, someone with shoulder pain typically develops an inappropriate firing pattern in one or both of their shoulders. The person is aware only of pain and clicking; but under most circumstances, does not understand why.

During my evaluation, the person is directed to first squeeze my hand and then squeeze and rotate the wrist against my resistance both internally and externally. These motions are all dependent on proper function in the shoulder joint and core muscles as well as a stable pelvis. I look for the person's shoulder to pop up or elevate, causing him to shrug his shoulder involuntarily as the body attempts to complete the task asked to perform.

This is invaluable as it immediately shows a mechanism of malfunction and poor coordination in the shoulder joint muscles. The effect is the recruitment of the neck and adjacent muscles in the region to assist in the movement. This is what causes the shoulder to pop up. These recruited muscles are not designed to assist in this activity, but activate when the firing pattern is poor, helping the person complete the action. The net effect is tightness and pain at and about the poorly firing joint mechanism.

I next look for tightness in the hips, in the abdominal muscles, in the deep pelvic muscles, and restrictions of movement at, or surrounding the shoulder girdle as tight shoulder joints are often restricted by muscles in the lower body. I further confirm that there are no other structural problems in the shoulder joint such as a torn glenoid labrum, generalized instability or tight joint capsule. If the additional problems I am ruling out exist, it reduces the likelihood of a favorable outcome and other measures may need to be taken.

When I am comfortable that all the muscles and tissues disrupting normal function are identified then tools such as myofascial release, Graston Technique® and other methods are used to work out the muscular problems, adhesions and restrictions. Then the joint is retested to see if it is firing better with less recruitment in the muscles surrounding the shoulder. If it functions better, other muscles that are keeping the shoulder from working appropriately are treated until an acceptable level of coordination and strength improvement in the area is reached.

After a more appropriate level of function is achieved, the patient reports on their next visit how they feel and I re-evaluate how they are doing using the same procedures. If I correctly identified the dysfunctional tissues, the person returns the following day noting an overall improvement. They show less recruitment, greater strength and less pain.

The process continues as we eliminate the various mechanical issues that caused the problem. Only when the area is showing a consistent improvement in strength and coordination and can offer significantly more resistance with less pain upon testing the region is an exercise and weight training regimen designed to strengthen the area to improve function more quickly.

This differs markedly from what happens typically in the field. Generally, practitioners tell patients to exercise *before* the problem region can tolerate it. This results in pain and further function loss due to improper firing patterns left uncorrected. It makes little sense adding weight to an area that has difficulty with gravity.

The philosophy and treatment method described is also very different from the trendy and faddish passive care phenomena consisting of electronic muscle stimulation, ultrasound, stretching of the muscles and other exotic, but less effective methods directed only toward the site of pain (and not necessarily the problem) commonly seen today in many offices. While these modalities of treatment offer temporary relief, my experience is that manual methods offer faster and more reliable long-term outcomes.

This is an uncomplicated explanation of the process of diagnosis and treatment of the shoulder. You can see that it is clearly a non-invasive and low-tech process of elimination. Identify causative factors, create a working diagnosis for the day, act upon it, re-test and then re-evaluate during the follow-up visit.

When there is sufficient improvement, exercises are added to further strengthen the area. The method is scientific and predictable. If there is no predictable progression of improvement within a reasonable period of time (three weeks), as the doctor I am either doing something wrong, I need to do something differently or there is a problem with stability within the joint that may require further testing and more aggressive intervention. Since the majority of people improve with this method of evaluation and treatment, many expensive diagnostic MRIs and similar evaluations are avoided, making care far more cost effective.

Treating the causes of shoulder problems properly improves many other chronic conditions simply because shoulder problems are usually secondary to the pelvis, hip flexors, leg muscles and gait cycle. Since these areas are addressed in the treatment of the shoulder issue, many other patient complaints of less immediate importance improve or disappear.

For instance, after treatment, as there is now little or no muscular recruitment, the neck, shoulder blade and forearm and wrist articulations work better and are less likely to develop future pain and joint damage. These could have been future problems that would have presented themselves if we did not treat the mechanical cause of the shoulder problem. In other words, you fix the problem and a bunch of problems resolve or significantly improve, including the ones that are not yet symptomatic. Go figure!

It is important to note that most health care practitioners are not trained to recognize dysfunctional movement patterns that cause inappropriate function resulting in pain about the neck and shoulder joint.

Most people know one of two things when they visit me; either they feel good or they don't. Patients look to someone like me to figure out why they are in pain and to make it go away. They are and will remain oblivious as to why they are in pain unless someone understands it well enough to show them and explain it to them coherently in terms they can understand.

The fact is that while we all share common traits, we are all built differently; and that makes things a little messy, if not a little difficult. Think about it. All cars share common traits, too. They have a body, an engine, tires, shocks, lights, steering mechanism, a fuel source, a way to go and a way to stop and they all come with owner's manuals for maintenance and repair specific to the make, model and year.

Unfortunately, the human body does not come with an owner's manual for your particular body style- your make and model. Unless someone can show you why you are in pain and why it happens to you in a way you can understand, you will always think that the problem one time was that my shoulder went bad, another time it was my neck. Or, that I have a bad knee, weak ankles, problem-prone wrists, etcetera, etcetera, and etcetera, all because nobody connected the dots for you.

Admittedly, it is difficult to be objective about one's self regarding multiple symptoms processes. It is even more difficult since our health care system leads us to believe that each symptom is a tendonitis, a myositis, a herniated disc, a meniscus tear, or some other discrete issue. Instead, our current system offers medical niche experts and specialists who gladly take care of each of these symptoms for you independently and unquestioningly, as if they are all separate and discrete entities.

These "experts" prescribe medications and injections to decrease poorly understood inflammation and pain. Then, following years of neglect, they recommend surgery to correct the symptom of a bony impingement or arthritic problem; a problem that developed from a global dysfunction within the joints of your body, which was sadly caused because they diagnosed and treated your pain symptomatically instead of functionally.

You are likely find that as one symptom goes away another symptom appears in another area of your body. You learn to tolerate the other problems that only become painful on occasion with some sort of activity. This is most common and noticeable as people age and, unfortunately, they mistakenly attribute it to aging. Furthermore, the myth is often substantiated by family members, other lay people and even your doctor.

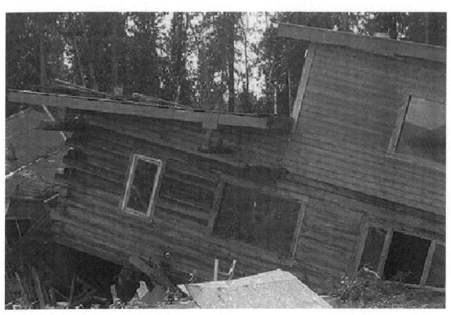

Treating symptoms instead of function is like using mud to shore up the sides of the building with a bad foundation. Over time, the building will experience major structural damage even with the mud, since the true problem of the foundation was never addressed. Only by fixing the foundation, can you truly repair the problems in the building. The same is true for the human body. That is why an enlightened practitioner looks at the entire person, all the visual, mechanical and historical evidence he can collect and not just the person's symptoms.

> **Carpal Tunnel Syndrome** (CTS) is more common in women than it is in men, with more cases reported by people in their early forties. Studies show that about ten percent of the adult population is "at risk" for CTS.

A great example of a consequence of misinterpreting shoulder pain is a patient who came into our office frustrated with his previous practitioner. This patient was experiencing chronic pain throughout his body. His main complaint, however, was carpal tunnel syndrome (CTS), or median nerve impingement at the wrist.

The classic definition of CTS based on our current health care paradigm is a condition commonly described as a medical condition where the median nerve at the wrist is compressed, causing pain, a sensation of tingling, pricking or numbness, and muscle weakness in the forearm and hand.

Our current system of evaluation as used by most physicians takes a global mechanical dysfunction and describes the end result which is tingling, numbness and pain that is presumed to be from overuse, or repetitive work. They then give it a name that describes the symptomatic functional result, which in this case is Carpal Tunnel Syndrome.

Recommended by many credible sources to reduce wrist pain by preventing certain motions, this patient was wearing splints on his wrists at night. Common to the condition, the patient had limited external rotation of both forearms and restricted extension of both wrists.

His previous doctors looked only at his wrist because their training assumes that this must be the cause. They did not look elsewhere for the cause of the problem as their training did not teach them to do so. They did not see that he had moderate to severe foot overpronation, a significant tightness in his core muscles, in his legs and in his hip flexors, and that he could not raise his arms over his head because these areas were not symptomatic. Additionally, the patient suffered chronic knee soreness, headaches, and aching in both shoulders.

This patient liked to play guitar (something I can personally relate to) and had difficulty playing because his arms would not allow him to get into the proper posture for positioning his fingers on the neck of the guitar. He did not become truly concerned until he was told he needed surgery after a nerve conduction test (NCV) which tests for nerve entrapment and is typically used to convince people of the need for carpal tunnel surgery.

In just three months from walking into my office he was comfortably raising his arms over his head, the pain in his legs improved, his overall flexibility increased, and he was playing the guitar with greater ease without having surgery.

What was the secret? A combination of hands-on, low-tech solutions addressed multiple issues.

First, I prescribed shoe inserts to correct his foot posture and improve his body symmetry.

Second, I applied myofascial release treatment and Graston Technique® to the patient's muscles. Spinal and rib manipulations were used to restore normal mobility in his affected joints; and finally exercise was encouraged to the degree to which it could be tolerated.

Upon discharge, mechanically speaking, he was able to lift weights without pain. He was getting stronger in his lower body and the symptoms in his upper back and neck had improved markedly. Overall, his sense of wellbeing had greatly improved.

In addition to experiencing a better functioning body and an improved quality of life, he now understood how his body works and saw many of his traits (inherited traits) in his twin children. He understood what could happen when a person ignores body style. He is now more likely to be sure that his children, too, wear inserts because he now understands the consequences of body style, and he knows they will feel and function much better when wearing them.

He also better understands that certain symptoms in the shoulders, neck, hands or other parts of the body have a reason. He knows now that pain does not usually "just happen," and that there are ways to improve the way you feel, function and age.

It is really very simple: better function ultimately causes less wear and tear on the body and provides a better experience and quality of life as you age.

We are first beginning to quantify the cost to the health care system of someone who only knows they have pain, covers it up with medications and tries applying numerous therapies to the painful parts. Ignorance of function and a lack of appropriate education about preventive measures such as foot orthotics results in surgeries later in life that simply address the symptoms and do not treat the cause. Knowledge results in aging gracefully, with less pain and a better quality of life. Better overall health requires fewer healthcare resources and, therefore, costs less while the person enjoys fewer physical limitations and disabilities later in life.

Quite simply, a person with an asymmetrical body style and foot flare who takes poor care of himself when he is young becomes a likely candidate for new hips, knees and other joints that wear out from supposed over use.

Today, a person in his forties, whose parents took action thirty years ago to understand how body style determines function, is less likely to experience the need for part replacements and chronic pain medication as he ages because his body simply works better.

What is the lesson here? Take the time and evaluate your children now. Years ago, we were less knowledgeable about body mechanics. Today, we have no excuse!

The average life span increases by a couple of years every decade. I am betting you know of more people in their eighties today than you knew twenty years ago. That means the chances that you will live well into your eighties or longer is increasing too. Take action now when you are in your twenties, your thirties and your forties to understand your body style and take a preventive, non-surgical, non-invasive course of activity that can greatly enhance the quality of your life as you age, and save you some anxiety, time and money along the way.

Elbow, Arm and Hand Pain Syndromes and Symptoms of Numbness

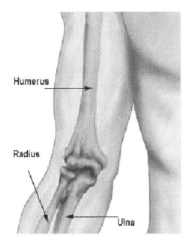

Humerus

Radius

Ulna

When the shoulder functions poorly, the elbow, wrist, thumb and other digits are likely to develop problems due to strain and recruitment into those areas.

The upper kinetic chain (shoulder-elbow-wrist-digits) is affected by both the angle at which the shoulder works and the tightening of the tissues surrounding the forearm and elbow from recruitment of other muscles surrounding the shoulder thereby causing the shoulder to function less efficiently.

Problems in the forearm are aggravated when the external rotation of the shoulder becomes markedly reduced; causing secondary straining into the elbow and forearm, and then finally the wrist, which eventually affects finger function.

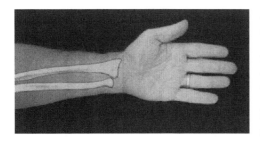

This area is unique because the elbow and the wrist are both governed by two multiple moveable joints made up of the ulna and radius. These bones are shaped to allow free rotation of the forearm at the elbow and freedom of movement at the wrist in many different directions. This unique design gives the human hand fine motor function manipulation ability, allowing the hand to manipulate things in a unique and exact way. Without this design feature, our arm dexterity would be limited and we would be forced to use our bodies differently.

Experiencing any impairment in these mechanisms can lead to nerve entrapments and other physical limitations because of the altered way in which you would have to adapt to the new limitation.

For example, a patient had the misfortune of fracturing his wrist at the ulna bone, which is on the side of the pinky. His orthopedist, looking to stabilize a painful injury, believed it was in the patient's best interest to fuse the ulna (the long bone in the forearm that attaches at the wrist most near where your pinky begins) by using a piece of metal to the other wrist bones in the area with the result of totally immobilizing the ulna bone.

Now the patient is no longer able to perform simple movements like turning a doorknob without engaging his shoulder abnormally to make up for the lost mobility at the wrist and elbow.

Over time, the side effect of this well-intentioned, poorly chosen course of action was near total numbness into half of his hand, pinky and forth finger from chronic overuse and adhesion of the localized structures to the ulna nerve.

More about the patient and treatment in moment; First, a little background to help you understand the severity of the situation beyond a fused ulna as secondarily he developed muscular and nerve adhesions in his shoulder affecting his arm, hand, shoulder and neck muscles.

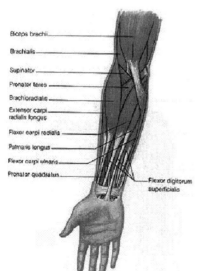

When the shoulder tightens resulting in a loss of proper rotation and leverage, it causes recruitment of the biceps, triceps, brachialis (the muscles in the upper arm that attach to the elbow region) pronator teres, pronator quadratus as well as other muscles that occupy the front of the forearm (muscles that rotate the forearm down, stabilize it and allow our fingers to make a fist). The resulting tightness strains the joints to which they attach.

As these muscles attempt to compensate for shoulder instability and the resulting loss of mechanical advantage, the tissues the surrounding myofascia tighten.

Between these muscles lie the ulna and radial nerves, which over time can become entrapped along their paths by the constant straining, tightening and healing of their adjacent muscles during daily activities. Poor upper kinetic chain coordination (arm, wrist and shoulder) causes muscles to overwork and strain as they compensate for shoulder insufficiency caused by improper core, lower kinetic chain joint and muscular function.

Poor muscular coordination not only creates less leverage when attempting to perform your desired movement (opening a door for instance), the muscles become overloaded as they attempt to make the movement you desire without the other parts of your body assisting and stabilizing in the way that is expected.

The chronic recruitment in these tissues causes the area to continue to tighten over time unless something is done to improve functionality.

When the biceps and triceps tighten abnormally because of poor shoulder torque and firing, the long axis movements of both the ulna and radius are also affected. This ultimately can lead to restrictions of movement at the elbow and then too much movement at the wrist. This ultimately can cause wrist pain, carpal tunnel syndrome, hand numbness issues, tendonosis inside and outside of the elbow (also known as golfer's and tennis elbow), and other conditions such as trigger fingers as the muscles in the forearm become shortened and tightened, causing adhesions along the tendon sheaths that become hung up along their path.

Additionally, problems like thumb pain, pain in the wrist when using a computer mouse, chronic shoulder blade tightness and numbness in the hand and arm at night can occur in other areas of the hand, with arthritic changes over time and chronic thumb pain.

Current solutions include bracing of the hands at night, ergonomic computer mouse peripherals, chairs, trays and other devices that attempt to reduce stress on the body. Many people rely on tennis elbow braces to relieve elbow pain during certain sports and some have the area treated by a massage therapist.

Clinical solutions to address the issues include physical therapy that may attempt treatment using ultrasound and other therapies such as massage and exercises to strengthen the forearm. If that does not work, more aggressive treatments and evaluations including surgeries and nerve transpositions are considered[74].

Even though these methods are discussed in the current literature, the validity of many of these procedures have often not been proven satisfactorily, and the long term results are less than compelling because they attempt to re-engineer the region so it works differently than it was intended[75]. There are better, more reliable options available. However, depending on whom the patient visits, those options may never be realized because of the personal bias or knowledge of the consulting physician[76].

Back to our patient; when I first saw the patient, he had minimal grip strength and a total lack of sensation in the lateral side of his hand. When I completed my care to enhance the functionality of the area, he exhibited improved grip strength. He was able to use his last two fingers to grip. He enjoyed a better range of motion in his neck and shoulders, and had better overall function.

As I monitored his progress during monthly follow-ups, the patient continued to exhibit a loss of feeling in his pinky. However, overall there was much more sensation and strength, primarily due to the work performed on the forearm, pelvis and shoulder girdle. Eventually, we discussed having the doctor remove the metal bar in his wrist to allow for more mobility if possible.

This example clearly shows how the loss of rotation in the forearm can have dire consequences because of the impairment it causes in a human being. There is a reason our upper body adapted to allow the type of motion we evolved in our arms. There is a reason that reengineering what nature has perfected over time by natural selection is not necessarily a good idea. To put it another way, function follows form and your form will adapt to unnatural functional changes, as in the case of welding two bones together with a metal plate.

Unfortunately, when someone experiences a fracture in multiple places and the patient is in considerable pain, the doctor has to make a decision as to how to get the area to function as normally as possible when it heals. Could full range of motion have been a workable alternative for this injury? Nobody can say for sure. However, great care must be taken when modifying kinetic chains. It makes sense to restore function to the entire mechanism, not just the part that is injured or in pain. While this is not always possible, ultimately, function should always be restored as much as possible in a way that assures that the patient has an acceptable level of function not only now, but in years to come.

What is glaringly missing in the traditional thought process is the search for the cause in areas other than those that have obvious symptoms! Notice, bracing, surgeries, and most rehab will look at the arm and wrist where the symptoms are present. What about the rest of the body that often creates the problem?

I will say it again. The kinetic chains are the problem. Pain, disability and numbness are usually the end product.

The public, accustomed to symptoms being considered and addressed, does not generally know the difference unless they have been educated appropriately. Most people who have not read this book will continue to believe that stuff just happens and that pain can be taken care of by treating the area that hurts, or with a medication of some sort, which will offer relief. If you are reading this book, consider yourself one of the few educated, armed and able to seek out appropriate care.

The True Cause of Painful and Numb Wrists, Hands and Fingers

Upon evaluation, I look at the patient, assess his body style, and then look at his symptoms. Through a functional evaluation, I follow the lower kinetic chains first and see how they are affecting the pelvis and the hip flexors. When body asymmetry is the cause, these areas are usually involved.

The next step is to check the core muscles and range of motion of the shoulders on the involved side(s). Tight core muscles make it difficult to raise the arms up, either laterally or in front. This causes chronic straining of the shoulder muscles with recruitment of the shoulder blade musculature since the shoulder has to work at an inefficient angle. When this occurs, the person loses the ability to rotate the arm externally, which in turn causes a tightening of the biceps and triceps in the arm. As a result, the person may also experience neck tightness since many of these same muscles are involved in moving the neck and upper back region.

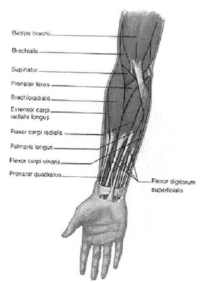

Biceps brachii
Brachialis
Supinator
Pronator teres
Brachioradialis
Extensor carpi radialis longus
Flexor carpi radialis
Palmaris longus
Flexor carpi ulnaris
Pronator quadratus
Flexor digitorum superficialis

If tight, these muscles restrict mobility at the elbow, usually with external rotation. However, internal rotation may also be involved as well. This restriction, in turn, causes tightness from chronic strain in the muscles that are below the elbow, including the pronator teres, brachialis and other forearm muscles.

It is common for these muscles with the surrounding fascia to attach via fascial adhesion to the median and ulna nerves. Repeated inflammation and healing adhesions with a loss of oxygen to the tissues causes the region to become tighter and more scarred over time. This mechanism was explained in the diagram of Dr. Leahy's Cumulatively Injury Cycle

These adhesions often cause numbness in the hand and fingers and are commonly confused with carpal tunnel syndrome, a condition that results from a tightening of the carpal ligament, which crosses at the wrist.

The condition impinges on the muscles, blood vessels and nerves that go through the carpal ligament into the hand creating pain, numbness and other symptoms.

The result is a number of elbow and forearm conditions including medial and lateral epicondylitis (both are forms of tendon problems resulting from tight forearm musculature), and numbness into the first two fingers or last finger due to nerve entrapments (often confused by many health care providers with carpal tunnel syndrome).

As I follow my evaluation into the wrist, I look for restricted movement of the wrist bones (carpal bones), radius and ulna at the wrist (the two forearm bones designed to allow for rotation in the forearm as well as flexibility at the wrist in a normal functioning arm end here). Restricted mobility in those joints is a result of tightening of the elbow musculature (biceps, triceps, and brachialis).

I then check to see if I can bring the arm into full extension with the palm up and extended without tissue or joint restriction or pain. Someone with true carpal tunnel syndrome will not fully be able to extend the arm and wrist because of the restrictions up the kinetic chain due to the tightening of the muscles, connective tissue and tendons.

I then check the thumb for entrapments or restrictions. If there are entrapments, there will typically be pain with forced motion. I check the other hand digits for signs of tendons that may have become entrapped in the palmar fascia connective tissue that can result in ganglions (painful fluid filled out pouching in a tendon) or in trigger fingers (the inability to extend fingers or the fingers feeling like they are getting stuck).

Following this painful kinetic road, you now see that when the kinetic chains malfunction below in the lower leg they affect the upper body in a big way.

Too many people are finding that our health care system does not commonly train physicians and other health care providers to follow this type of train of thought.

After understanding how gait, foot posture, asymmetry and kinetic chains work, how can our current solutions that only seek to evaluate and treat via the symptom model be cost effective solutions? Over time, our health care systems budgets are exploding, as people get older. Is the aging populace really the problem? If we began to treat the mechanisms, rather than the symptoms from those mechanisms, in all probability, you would see a marked improvement in quality of life as people experience fewer problems because the problem rather than the symptoms are explored. Fewer problems as we age mean fewer expensive solutions, fewer doctor visits, fewer sleepless nights due to pain and healthier aging process.

Body style issues result in functional impairment and often-chronic pain. Most treatment regimens for the musculoskeletal system have varied results using our current system. Inter-reliability between practitioners (doctors coming to the same diagnosis) may not be as reliable as once thought to be acceptable, however it is the current basis for recommending care.

Other Hand and Finger involvement issues

Kinetic chain malfunction runs from the feet through the knees, hips and shoulders and affects the hands as well. Once the forearm is involved, the finger flexors and extensors can also develop problems due to loss of blood flow in the anterior compartment (the front of forearm) or the posterior compartment of the forearm because the outer structures have tightened.

In this diagram, the muscles in the forearm (darker) end with the tendons (lighter) and then into the carpal tunnel (ligamentous band across the wrist bones) into the wrist.

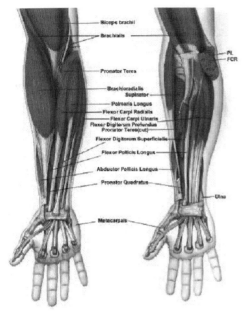

Problems in the forearm can eventually lead to problems in the hand that include but are not limited to trigger finger, ganglions, contractures (shortening and tightening of tissues making them unusable and inflexible), thumb pain as well as other painful hand syndromes. Many of these hand problems that people experience are the result of tendon malfunction, which occurs with muscular tightening in the forearm resulting from malfunction of other areas of the kinetic chain.

When muscles become tighter and less compliant, the forces placed on tendons increase markedly, creating chronic injury and re-injury cycles, which make the tissue less pliable and brittle, eventually creating a painfully chronic condition known as tendonosis (a scarred brittle tendon that readily develops more micro tears from regular use).

Typical movements can make the region very sore and painful, and even disabling over time. Unless you do something to improve the function of the muscles and tendons, and correct the malfunction that created the situation, you will likely experience chronic pain or acute pain with certain activities that most people can do easily. People with significant problems often visit rheumatologists, take many drugs for symptom relief or are under pain management care. Perhaps, they need other options of types of health care providers on a more consistent basis.

Effective treatment should include Myofascial Release and Graston Technique®. Graston tools are incredibly effective because they work well on tendons and because one of the tools is smaller than the fingers, allowing easier access to involved tissue adhesions in hard to get at regions such as the base of the thumb and in between digits. It works wonderfully when the palmar fascia (connective tissue in the palm) becomes tight resulting in stiffness, and tendon entrapment, which can lead to other painful conditions of the hand and digits. Trigger fingers are also treatable using Graston Technique® and is an alternative to surgical intervention.

In most cases where the forearm muscles have shortened, the shoulder joint is tight and cannot extend properly or rotate outward. This, as you have learned, often originates in the feet, legs and pelvis.

Your health care provider needs to evaluate the entire kinetic chains and, regardless of your specific symptom, consider lower extremity issues before treating your problem. Right now, few providers work this way. However, if we ever wish to make our health care system more effective and productive, our educational systems need to fully embrace and teach the idea of treating cause and make a real effort to reeducate the many health care providers who currently do not think this way.

Looking Past Your Symptoms

The Case of the Finger and the Foot

Imagine walking into your doctor's office unable to pour a glass of water or comfortably hold a cup of tea and walking out of the office a short time later absent the concern. Here's the story.

A female patient called and complained of right hand pain into her thumb and index finger with trigger finger in the right hand. She stated that the finger always clicks and she decided to schedule an appointment with me after hearing about Graston Treatment® on the evening news.

While taking the patient's history, I noticed her right shoulder leaned forward and her right foot turned out, indicating foot overpronation with foot flare. So, I asked about other problems in her hips. You should know that hip issues were not a part of the history she provided. Then, when I asked about her shoulder (also not part of the offered history), she said she experiences chronic right shoulder and neck pain that has worsened over the years, but that she "tolerates it."

The patient stated she was under the care of a chiropractor who saw her monthly for her lower back pain and that she had polio as a child that affected her right side and left her with a right dropped foot. A dropped foot is a condition where a person cannot lift her toes up, causing irregularity in their walking ability. In this patient's case, the dropped foot was attributed to post polio syndrome.

Further questioning revealed that she never adopted foot orthotics because they never fit in her shoes properly. The prosthetic lab did, however, make her a foot assist to help keep the foot up and prevent the toes from getting caught when walking. She refused to wear the assist because it would not allow her to wear her regular shoes.

> Note: The patient's main complaint concerned her hand. She had no idea that there may be a relationship between the right foot flare, right shoulder, and lower back pain on the left and chronic neck tightness.

Evaluation confirmed right foot drop, tortipelvis (pelvis was twisted), inability to raise the right shoulder due to adhesion inside the right shoulder joint as well as tightness in right abdominal muscles, psoas muscle and right erector spinae muscles. The patient was initially unable to grip my hand without excruciating pain in her right wrist. The patient also had moderate foot overpronation, more severe on the right.

Management on her first visit included myofascial release to quadratus lumborum and erector spinae bilaterally, right psoas, right lower trap, right subscapularis, right biceps and triceps and brachialis muscle.

Upon retesting patient's right hand grip strength, she was able to grip my right hand without pain and showed significantly greater grip strength.

The patient was given a small off-the-shelf (not custom made) foot orthotic. These fit in her shoe easily and solved the problem of the device not fitting her shoes.

I achieved the improvement in function in her hand because I did not treat her hand. The problem in her hand was the result, not the cause. I treated the cause. The cause was a dysfunctional foot and secondary body asymmetry, with torsion of the pelvis aggravated by neurological involvement from polio.

This patient arrived like most do believing that all her complaints were separate and distinct and were multiple pains and problems.

> Foot Orthotics are simply a brace that works while in your shoe.
>
> A foot orthotic that is not worn is ineffective.
>
> As a rule, I always try to find a way for the person to incorporate a foot orthotic easily into their lifestyle.

The patient walked out of the office with markedly less pain *everywhere* in her body and with the ability to grip things. Something she could not do previously without significant pain.

Most health care providers fall into the trap of evaluating and attempting to treat the symptoms though the problem is clearly functional in nature when you look at function and past the obvious symptoms.

Partly to blame (or maybe largely to blame) are the media stories and drug company advertising reinforcing the myth of symptoms being the problem. For example, if you have knee pain, you should take Nuprin®. For arthritis, take Excedrin®. Of course, the patient then asks the health care provider to find a solution to their symptom and even requests prescriptions for the pharmaceutical strength brand she saw on television that talked about the syndrome or medical condition and the drug that will alleviate it.

Many more health care providers are finding that patients come in just to request a particular medication for a set of symptoms they heard about in a commercial, since it sounds like the product will resolve their problem.

Patients begin to believe they have the disease they heard about and like their doctor, believe their pain is part of a disease process instead of understanding that their problems are a result of poor function. This is at the root of many chronic pain problems including myofascial pain syndrome.

Calling functional problems diseases and then treating them as if they are diseases only helps to strain joints. This contributes to the eventual break down that requires replacement when the joint becomes a source of disability and pain and is no longer functional.

This is clearly preventable. The era of back pain in Room 2, knee pain in Room 3, shoulder pain in Room 4 should change to the Gait-Related Issues in Rooms 2-4.

The Case of Restoring Bird Flipping Flexibility

Another patient read an article on Trigger finger and the Graston Technique®. When I met the patient, he showed me his middle finger, which was painful when I shook his hand. Moving the finger passively was excruciatingly painful. This had been going on for months, with the patient splinting the finger at night to keep it loose, without relief.

During consultation, the patient denied other problems. However, when he got up, he did so slowly due to back stiffness that he considered normal. Visually, I could see his left foot turned out and his left shoulder leaned in.

Tightness was noted in the left quadriceps, gluteal, psoas, pectoral muscles, bicep, triceps and pronator teres in the front of the forearm.

During the evaluation, the patient admitted going to the gym frequently, working through the pain, and more recently having some shoulder and neck tightness. Visually, the patient had tortipelvis, tightness in the core muscles, quadriceps, psoas, and subscapularis on the left side. Neck and lower back ranges of motion were restricted and the patient was only able to bend forward from the hips about 45 degrees. The patient was wearing worn-out foot orthotics prescribed from his previous chiropractor. However, he was wearing them in the wrong shoes (right orthotic in left shoe and visa versa).

> **Note:** Did you notice that I evaluated the entire body for what essentially was a hand problem on both patients? Both improved even though I never actually worked on their hands. They both had other sig nificant symptoms that did not seem important to them at the time but were indeed relevant to the long-term symptoms they were experiencing. This is why you want to find a doctor who looks past the obvious, understands the kinetic chains and human motion and can think outside the box.

Treatment included loosening up the muscles on the left side of his body to free up mobility in the left shoulder. The patient noticed a marked improvement in hand and finger flexibility, and was able to grip my hand without pain. He also noted a significant improvement in flexibility of his lower back when touching his toes.

To illustrate, let's use the example of opening a door. Most people think that to open a door, you grab the knob, turn and pull. You know. "It's all in the wrist."

Here is what really happens: We stabilize our pelvis, which stabilizes the shoulder and affects the position the shoulder assumes in the glenoid (the socket in which the humerus bone sits). We then use the shoulder to initiate arm movement and use the shoulder muscles to do most of the work.

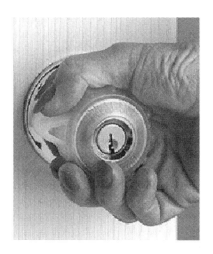

Secondarily, we use the arm for fine motor control. For detailed manipulation, we use the fingers and the wrist. When these mechanisms break down, we recruit and begin to use the shoulder and / or the elbow and the wrist as a prime mover. The net result is pain in the shoulder, elbow or wrist as the area becomes strained and the muscles and ligaments become sore and tighten from overload.

The Effect of Weight on the Human Frame

Obesity is an American epidemic. Not so long ago, we prepared our meal first by hunting and farming, then skinning the animal and then preparing the meal. My friend's father-in-law is fond of reminding the grandchildren that chopping wood was the first order of business every day. If they wanted to eat, they chopped wood.

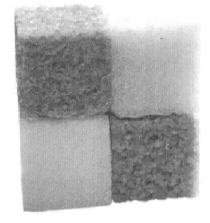

This took a huge amount of effort. We had smaller portioned meals. We ate at different intervals of time. We actually sat down. Our food was fresh and our vegetables were freshly picked and full of natural nutrients, which decrease over time as vegetables sit around in the supermarket.

Today, most of our food is pre-packaged or store purchased. Preparation may include the strenuous task of turning the dial and pressing the button on the microwave. There is not much effort and as a result, no fitness gain.

Instead, many of us rely on going to the gym or playing sports to get the exercise which years ago was achieved through walking, hunting, food preparation and just plain struggling to survive.

In American society, we have become accustomed to the larger portions of food and the high caloric meals with outrageous levels of simple carbohydrates that convert easily to sugar. Most Americans consume more than we burn with activity and, as a result have become larger and suffer from the many health problems that accompany the modern lifestyle. There is some evidence that slightly under-eating is actually healthier and causes the release of Leptins (http://en.wikipedia.org/wiki/Leptin), which help in weight regulation and possibly contribute to a longer lifespan.

The connection here is this: the large amount of weight on certain body styles creates chronic pain and prematurely damages the joints in the legs, back and spine. Many of us who are overweight and eat poorly have more medical problems that fuel the ever-escalating cost of health care[77]. Those countries that have begun to assimilate aspects of the American diet into their indigenous diets, like fast food, are finding their rates of heart disease, diabetes and other common American health issues are increasing along with their belt size[78]. Still, interestingly enough, not all overweight people have joint problems.

I believe that the main variant between overweight people who have problems versus those who do not is their body style, which can cause chronic pain. Whether you are thin or heavy, if you are built asymmetrically, the joint damage that can occur without the use of orthotics and treatment of the core muscles is very probable.

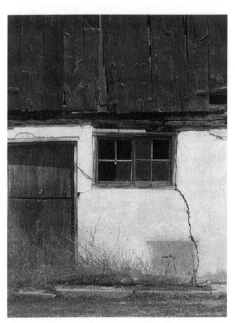

Those who lead active lives and those who are under stress are more likely to have problems if they are built asymmetrically and have feet that flare out with low or flat arches.

In these cases, people who are overweight are simply placing more weight on a frame that is inefficient and problematic to begin with.

Think of it this way. An overweight, asymmetrical body is similar to a two-story house with a badly poured foundation to which you decide to add an additional level. Over time, the foundation will be unable to support the added weight of the third floor. The house will start to show cracks and damage in a much worse and more pronounced way than when the home had only two floors.

Weight loss for someone with body style issues is essential. However, it can be quite painful for people with problems like this to tolerate exercise, especially at the beginning of their program.

You need only watch a few episodes of the television program "The Biggest Loser" to see the difficulty in moving a large body unaccustomed to exercise and de-conditioned. It is even more difficult for people who have mechanical issues created by body asymmetry. The results of movement and activity can be quite dramatic, not only in terms of weight loss but in the overall quality of life the person experiences.

The Road to Recovery, Weight Loss, Fitness and Better Health

Doctors advise people with weight issues to lose weight for their health; No argument there. Most major companies like Bristol Myers – Squibb and Johnson and Johnson, virtually in my backyard, have gyms in their complexes because they are aware of the studies declaring that fit employees are not only healthier, costing them less in health care payouts, but also perform better at their jobs. Many have collected statistics proving this assertion, finding that fit employees are more productive and have fewer days out of the office for health related problems.

Of course, it does not hurt that the gym is typically a non-taxable fringe benefit and that their healthcare carriers often provide discounts on insurance premiums for promoting use of the facilities.

Sounds terrific, right? Unfortunately, many of the people taking advantage of the gym benefit experience pain. Of course, a reasonable amount of pain at the beginning of a fitness program is not abnormal. Usually the first couple of workout sessions leave you sore due to delayed onset muscle soreness, a common but normal phenomenon during a first workout even if you are not overweight. You can read more about it at http://en.wikipedia.org/wiki/Delayed_onset_muscle_soreness.

However, if you have biomechanical problems, you not only feel sore, but likely hurt as you experience joint strain as well as muscle soreness. You may want to discontinue because the harder you push the more pain you experience.

I recommend biomechanical evaluations to everyone prior to beginning an exercise regimen; especially if they are overweight. Why; let me explain.

Most people are familiar with the family doctor doing a blood workup and checking their heart to assure them they are okay for exercise. Most people, however, do not consider the importance of a biomechanical evaluation as part of their pre-workout regimen.

Since most primary doctors specialize in looking at body organ systems problems and not the musculoskeletal system, a chiropractor, rehabilitation therapist, certified athletic trainer or professional with similar credentials could be more helpful when evaluating you for function.

This is important because painful conditions often appear when a poorly functioning region of the body is loaded with more weight and stress than is normally experienced during typical daily activities.

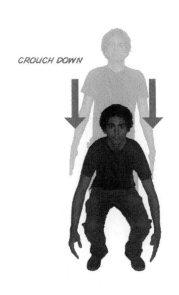

CROUCH DOWN

An evaluation of people thinking about beginning a workout regimen should include the following eight functional movement screens:

1. Check the feet and pelvis for asymmetry.
2. Balance on one leg, and then the other. Can they do this with a straight leg

for 30 seconds on either side? If they lose their balance while trying to perform this with the eyes open is a good indicator of a problem waiting to happen.

3. Can they touch their toes?

4. Is lateral bending and rotation at the waist and neck symmetrical?

5. Is rotation of the back and neck symmetrical?

6. Testing for mechanical advantage; Pushing against the healthcare provider's hands with their hands. (If the person pushes against the provider's hands with theirs, does the provider go back or does the patient? In other words, if the patient uses their body efficiently and has good leverage in this simple task, it usually indicates good shoulder and good core stability and function.)

7. Can they stand up with hands pressing lightly on their shoulders? (An inability to do this or having one shoulder dip is indicative of problems in the core muscles and bodies foundation. If one shoulder dips while they are attempting to get up, there is a strong likelihood they will experience problems as they load their body with exercises.)

8. One powerful, yet simple, final test is to have the patient perform a deep knee bend slowly. (I discovered long ago that if there are problems in the core muscles and there is poor symmetry and coordination, the person will lose their balance and may even fall over when trying to go down or get up. A typical sign of core trouble is the need to grab on to something as they crouch down or get up. An observer will also notice one hip dropping back while the other goes forward and the knee rolling in as the other rolls out as well.)

There may be other methods of functional movement evaluation, depending on the style of the evaluator that can help point out problems that are likely to occur and leave you in pain. Nevertheless, the above-mentioned have the Charschan seal of approval for consistent diagnosis.

If you cannot perform these tasks during the evaluation (typically, a number of these tests can be difficult)and you will need to address the asymmetry in your feet with orthotics. You will also need to address the muscular and joint issues by engaging a qualified therapist who understands body mechanics and is able to use myofascial release, Graston

Technique® or other methods to effectively treat the problems and enable you to function better against gravity.

Once these problems are identified and treated appropriately, you should be able to train without experiencing abnormal pain and instead greatly enhance your chance of embarking into a successful exercise regimen. Essentially, proper care will markedly improve the success of the rehabilitation process.

Pain is quite de-motivating. The ability to work out to enabling weight loss in the absence of pain, with the assistance of changes in your diet, is much more likely to enable you to make long-term changes in your lifestyle. The long-term goal with weight loss, of course, is better overall health, better overall fitness and a better quality of life.

Check out http://functionalmovement.com/SITE/. They are teaching and certifying health practitioners, rehabilitation providers, chiropractors, athletic trainers and other professionals in a proven method for finding functional weakness and improving potential outcomes with a better scientific method for finding faults in the human frame. These are the same faults that cause many people to experience chronic pain.

Nutritional Considerations

Other factors can be helpful in the management of lower back, neck and generalized joint pain. For example, nutritional supplementation following an acute injury to a lower back disc can improve the absorption of needed nutrients to the injured area and is thought to improve healing of the damaged tissues.

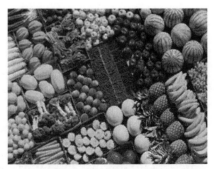

Nutritional substances and dietary regimens may decrease inflammatory responses. The following are known as anti-inflammation foods and are thought to help with chronic inflammatory problems:

Vegetables
Bell Peppers
Bok Choy
Broccoli
Broccoli Sprouts
Brussel Sprouts
Cabbage
Cauliflower
Chard
Collards
Fennel Bulb
Garlic
Green Beans
Breen Onions/ Spring Onions
Kale
Leeks
Olives
Spinach
Sweet Potatoes
Turnip Greens

Herbs & Spices
Basil
Cayenne Peppers/ Chilli Peppers
Cinnamon
Cloves
Cocoa (at least 70% cocoa chocolate)
Licorice
Mint
Oregano
Parsley
Rosemary
Thyme
Tumeric
Fish
Cod
Halibut
Herring
Oysters
Rainbow Trout
Salmon
Sardines
Snapper Fish
Tuna
Whitefish

Fruits
Acerola (West Indian) Cherries
Apples
Avocados
Black Currants
Blueberries
Fresh Pineapple
Guavas
Kiwifruit
Kumquats
Lemons
Limes
Mulberries
Oranges
Papaya
Raspberries
Rhubarb
Strawberries
Tomatoes

Nuts & Seeds
Almonds
Flaxseed/ Linseed
Hazelnuts
Sunflower Seeds
Walnuts

Oils
Avocado Oil
Extra Virgin Olive Oil

Drinks
Green Tea

You can read more about the concept at the Anabolic Labs web site - http://www.anaboliclabs.com/paCombatingChronicInflammation.aspx.

Before you start thinking that I am a shill, pushing nutritional supplementation and getting a piece of the action from the fishing industry you should understand by now that I am always skeptical when I read about ways to lubricate and rebuild cartilage, using supplementation as we age. Cartilage has poor vasculature and heals poorly. These methods may be helpful in relieving symptoms; however, I always go back to asking, "What caused the damage to the joint in the first place?"

More often than not, the seemingly innocent meniscus tear we attribute to the fall, the tennis game, picking up something and twisting does not just happen. A closer look shows poor body mechanics at work leading us eventually to the injury of that joint (s). Still, here are three more supplementation regimens that should be considered to help maintain joint health and during the healing phase of an injury.

Condroitin Sulfate and Glucosamine have been shown in some studies to be helpful because they are thought to help lubricate arthritic joints. Patients report to me that they find Condroitin Sulfate and Glucosamine helpful in managing joint pain due to arthritis[79].

The book, "The Arthritis Cure" by Jason Theodosakis, Brenda Adderly, and Barry Fox goes much more deeply into studies and the rationale for the usage of these substances, but the short of it is that since they are not harmful to the body, there is no harm in trying them.

When I injured a disc in my back (*yes, even chiropractors are subject to injury!*), a medical colleague who treats many athletes and is skilled with acupuncture suggested I try Bromelain to treat the disc inflammation.

Unlike most anti-inflammatory medications, Bromelain works at a relatively low dosage level and it works naturally. It is a proteolytic enzyme, which is a fancy way of saying meat tenderizer. Taking the recommended dosage of 400mg 2 - 3 times per day for the discomfort as needed, Bromelain took the edge off my pain. Vitamin B complex was part of the regimen and was helpful as well. Read more about Bromelain from Wikipedia at http://en.wikipedia.org/wiki/Bromelain.

Since our diets are not always well balanced, nutritional supplements can help fill in the gaps for us when we do not eat well. There is a lot of speculation about the positive effects of mega dosing large quantities of vitamins, however, and of course, that can get expensive. There is no solid evidence of which I am aware that suggests mega-dosing vitamins is any better for you than taking the multi-packs you can purchase in the health food store or Costco[80]. Taking these multi-packs three times per week should be sufficient to balance your dietary needs, even when compared to the more expensive one a day type vitamins of much lower dosage you can buy at your grocery store.

Nutritional health supplements may be a multi-billion dollar industry, but that is still just a fraction compared to pharmaceutical drug manufacturing.

Since the nutritional industry is neither nearly as well funded as the drug industry, nor as closely regulated, we may never see the level of research and oversight for nutritional products as compared to drugs that finally are approved and protected by patents.

Until we perform well funded, third party studies on the utilization of supplemental nutritional products and natural remedies, most of the information is likely to be based on the few studies that are available and anecdotal evidence.

Since most supplements used within reasonable levels are not harmful and may be beneficial to your overall health, there seems to be little to lose and much to gain by their regular usage.

Just keep in mind that while good nutritional habits may help, poor body mechanics will ultimately be the deciding factor in many painful conditions that prematurely wear down joints. Remember that as helpful as these dietary supplements may be, they cannot solve the mechanical process issues that cause joint degeneration and the painful conditions created by asymmetry and inefficient body mechanics.

Fixing more than your "Pain;" Fixing Your "Problem."

The health care system continues to teach doctors and therapists the disease model of evaluating back pain, neck pain, knee pain as well as other painful joints. By now, you should realize that since most often these problems begin at the feet and are a problem of body style, the bits and pieces resulting in chronic pain and disability as we age (knee pain, foot pain, toe pain, hip pain, etc) are simply yielding symptoms that are representative of the whole, but are not the problem.

Until the health care system, both in educational curriculum and in practice, is ready to change its tunnel-vision approach, the patient will continue to be handicapped, likely going from doctor to doctor looking for cures of a disease process at great expense since treating symptoms is simply not cost effective.

As the population ages, society finds itself rationing care due to the expense, rather than changing the paradigm that is creating a financial tsunami of healthcare costs because of problems that have been ignored for years. The functional basis of it all has never been addressed or universally understood. However, as you now know, what we put off today affects us more severely tomorrow with pain and a diminished quality of life.

It is time to take matters into your own hands. Find a practitioner who is holistic; one who looks outside the current health symptom-disease care box, and you will find someone most capable of understanding why you are in pain; someone who can look for and find real solutions that get you out of pain, and, in many cases, improve other health problems you didn't know were related.

Structural problems often cause neurological problems and somatic disorders, which can affect or mimic problems in organ systems.

For example, many common stomach complaints are actually of musculoskeletal origin. It is a fact that most upper and lower GI tests come back negative. Unfortunately, stomach complaints and the probability of muscular involvement are hardly ever diagnosed because patients are instead placed on medications based on their symptoms, and then tested with upper and lower GI and other procedural evaluations. Furthermore, doctors are incentivized to do more procedures and less evaluation because performing procedures pays better.

I recently treated a patient with stomach complaints. She was taking medication to relieve the discomfort and not sure if the medication was helping. She also had a pain in her shoulder blade. Upon evaluation, her pelvis was distorted. I worked on the muscles in the pelvis and her stomach symptoms subsided. She never needed medication. Had her gastro-intestinal doctor had some knowledge of the musculoskeletal system, she would never have needed the tests or the medication. Her doctor would have clearly seen there was a problem with her lower back. This story is actually is quite common.

By now, you should have a basic understanding of how kinetic chain malfunction causes leg, lower and upper back symptoms. The only logical path to resolving mechanical problems of the musculoskeletal system is to undo the poor mechanical function that created the problem in the first place. This differs from the disease based flow chart approach of treating pain with medication, exercise, deductive therapy, and diagnostics such as an MRI.

If the healthcare system treated you correctly, one practitioner could have evaluated, treated and released you; and you would feel a great long lasting improvement in your condition (providing there is not a situation providing neurological compromise).

Further, you would probably check back with this practitioner periodically over the years because you have begun to understand that your condition is likely an inherited trait. You have also begun to recognize that you may have the tendency to tighten up over time and require what is a legitimate well care, or maintenance care visit.

This is no different, really, than the care people seek from their dentist to assure their teeth stay healthy. Establishing a long-term relationship with this kind of health care practitioner will improve your quality of life.

When you are properly rehabilitated in your legs, back and other involved and recruited areas, and you wear properly fitting foot orthotics as needed which can vastly improve the way you walk and your overall body symmetry and structure, your need for ongoing care should be minimized greatly.

Where can you find a doctor like that?

Most people who go to doctors for a problem would like to be able to go to one place to get their problem resolved. It is efficient and is more likely to resolve your joint related problem than when you are evaluated by one doctor, tested by another, sent to a third for treatment, evaluated again in a few weeks, and if not better, being sent for more tests, which is currently the norm in our overspecialized health care system.

It is a blatant, shameless plug, but, if you are tired of being treated like a meat ping-pong ball and are serious about finding a one-stop doc, try a local chiropractor. Having read this book, you know the kind of philosophy he needs to have. You will know if he is the kind of doctor who can help.

In our chiropractic office, we look at the body as a whole. Sure, we are huge proponents of the effect body style, feet, and your core have on health; so we evaluate the joints, work on the musculature and toward establishing symmetry. We are a first contact health care provider similar to your primary care doctor. However, our point of view is different because the health care paradigm from which we work is different.

If you are uncomfortable with that, you should at least seek out a practitioner who looks past the obvious to resolve lower back pain issues. You now know why back pain is a gait issue. Care and evaluation that ignores the gait process is risking ignoring the true cause of why you are in pain; and the resulting care will likely reflect this with mediocre results or temporary relief rather than a long-term solution.

Those of you who have experienced back, neck, shoulder, foot or knee treatment that yielded either short-term results or an exacerbation from the treatment regimen understand the frustration of pain and disappointment when a promising course of treatment fails to help you get a great result. You deserve a doctor and course of treatment that can help.

Final Thoughts... For Now.

When we are in pain we often lose sight of the relationship between cause and effect because in addition to the physical impairment, pain has such a high emotional impact on our lives. It affects how we sleep, our relationships, how we manage in a social gathering, and how much pain each individual believes they can tolerate varies before requiring help.

As a consumer of health care, you owe it to yourself to find the right people for your health care team. You need to be sure your health care providers are willing to speak with each other and work on the same team; Your team.

Our current health care system is disjointed. Most painful conditions are not from the internal organs or from a life threatening conditions or disease processes as many people fear. Many people undergo numerous and unnecessary tests ordered by their doctor who is just trying to rule out disease as a cause, while covering themselves and trying to avoid malpractice if, on the very small chance they miss something life threatening. Most of these tests are negative for disease processes and quite costly by design.

Often, many types of pain symptoms originate in the musculoskeletal system.

If true emergency or life threatening problems are rare and most of these symptoms exist in the musculoskeletal system, a musculoskeletal workup should be protocol before running expensive tests.

Think of the cost savings to the health care system when your doctor, through manual evaluation is able to figure out why you are in pain and avoid the cost and planning of many of these tests.

Think of the speed, accuracy and lower cost of an effective treatment prescribed by a physician who understands function and is capable of performing a manual evaluation. There is a reason patient satisfaction is 25% higher for chiropractors than primary care physicians for treatment of musculoskeletal conditions!

The body, in its own way, tries to make you aware when something is not right. Listen to your body. It is doing its best to help itself and preserve you by using your survival instincts. You should have health care providers that are willing to speak with you and guide you to solutions that are sensible and helpful. You should be suspicious of many of the press releases and special reports on the news about new drugs, new miracle cures, and advances in health care. Often it is marketing, disguised as news.

Always be careful with new medications because even though your health care providers recommend them, current history has shown many of them are not as safe as older, tested medications with a history and track record. Many newer prescription pharmaceuticals are regularly removed from the market for safety reasons and further testing.

The bottom line is that all drugs have side effects and because of their nature cannot improve body mechanics. To use them for painful situations that have a basis in mechanical problems is like putting sawdust in the oil of your car to silence a serious problem in your engine. The sound may go away but the mechanical problem will eventually destroy your engine.

Getting to the true cause of the problem is the only reasonable way of improving function and resolving a problem.

Now, go forth armed with knowledge and questions to ask so you can live a healthier and happier life, longer.

-Dr. Bill Charschan

Exercise Bonus Section!

This section covers specific musculoskeletal issues and exercises used in my office patient care. As simple as these are, a reason my patients complete their course of rehabilitation, you should check with your physician if you have any question regarding the safety of pursuing these activities. Just remember to ask an enlightened practitioner!

If you would like to download and print out a larger version of each exercise with easy to follow pictures, please visit www.backfixer1.com/bookexercises. You will need to register to receive the key code to unzip the file.

Helpful Exercises for the Lower Back and Legs

When your body functions well, recovery from activity is generally fast. When your body functions poorly, you can be sore for days. Those who regularly work out at the gym should please pay attention here. If the pelvis is unstable due to gait issues that have not been properly addressed there is little point training the upper body because it will overwork and recruit in other poorly affiliated muscles causing marked soreness in the upper body, too. Simply put pelvic stability and symmetry is necessary for upper body strength and power.

Many people want to do things for themselves. This chapter reviews some basic exercises that our patients use to improve on their own while under care. It is important to note that these exercises will help tone the areas in question.

Another self-help regimen I commonly recommend (I almost cannot believe I am putting this in print) is the WII Fit, which has a virtual trainer, a computerized athletic trainer that is quite effective at toning up the mid-section of your body. It is both challenging and fun to do and I can state from personal experience that it works.

Roman Chair Exercises are quite helpful as well. A roman chair can be purchased inexpensively on line and is quite strong and stable. It is a great way of strengthening the lower back region. You can follow the instructions on the sheet.

Lower Back and Core Strengthening Exercises

Modified lower back extensions performed on the Roman Chair. ☐

These exercises when done as directed will strengthen the lower and mid back as well as the posterior neck muscles. From the position 1 (a), position you hands as shown (b). Slowly, feeling each spinal segment, lift your body. When you reach position 2 (c), move your hands across your chest as shows (d).

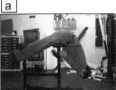 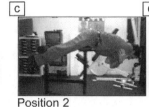

Position 1

As you continue to extend your back, you will reach neutral position 3 (body perpendicular to the floor) you place your hands behind your neck (f) and bring your neck into full extension (e). You will then slowly descend back down into position 1 and repeat. Begin with 6-8 repetitions and work toward 20-25 in one set.

Position 2 ☐

Exercises for lower back postural muscles (Erector Spinae)

These exercises are performed laying down on the floor with a small ball (beach ball e.g..). Lay on back with knees bent, making sure lower back is pressed against floor. Push knees into ball against wall as shown by tensing lower back muscles on side of the ball. Hold sustained contraction for 10 seconds. Increase to 50-60 seconds over a two to three week period.

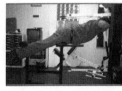

Position 3

Exercises for abdominal muscles on Roman Chair ☐

These exercises are performed with your buttock sitting over the pad on the roman chair and your feet under the rests on the chair. Allow your body to go into as much extension as tolerated (a).

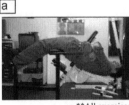 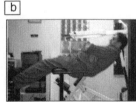

Slowly bring your body up until it reaches approximately 60 degrees (b). Then slowly go down to original position (a) again. Repeat initially for 4-6 reps and work toward 20-25 in one set.

**All exercises on this page to be performed every other day.

Other exercises helpful for the lower back are hip extensions, lateral leg raises, proprioceptive balancing exercises to retrain the leg neurologically and muscularly balance the leg and hip, and simple exercises to strengthen the shins and calves.

Lower Kinetic Chain Retraining Exercises

The first two exercises are to be performed daily. You will begin these standing on one leg straight. When you can do this without shaking too much for 30 seconds on each leg, then perform an additional 30 seconds daily with eyes closed. Then as this improves, do it with the leg bent and then with the leg bent, eyes closes for a total of 2 minutes on each leg. This can take up to 3 months or more to achieve the appropriate level of streingth and balance. **Be sure to balance from the hips, not the knee.**

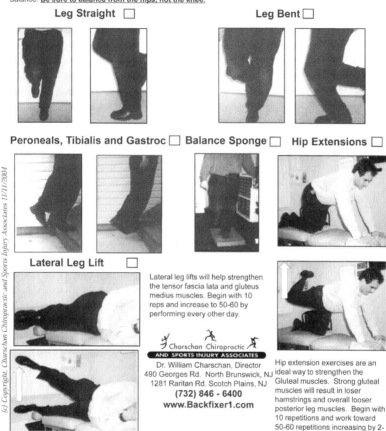

Leg Straight ☐   **Leg Bent** ☐

Peroneals, Tibialis and Gastroc ☐   **Balance Sponge** ☐   **Hip Extensions** ☐

Lateral Leg Lift ☐

Lateral leg lifts will help strengthen the tensor fascia lata and gluteus medius muscles. Begin with 10 reps and increase to 50-60 by performing every other day.

Charschan Chiropractic
AND SPORTS INJURY ASSOCIATES
Dr. William Charschan, Director
490 Georges Rd. North Brunswick, NJ
1281 Raritan Rd. Scotch Plains, NJ
(732) 846 - 6400
www.Backfixer1.com

Hip extension exercises are an ideal way to strengthen the Gluteal muscles. Strong gluteal muscles will result in loser hamstrings and overall looser posterior leg muscles. Begin with 10 repetitions and work toward 50-60 repetitions increasing by 2-4 every other day as tolerated.

(c) Copyright, Charschan Chiropractic and Sports Injury Associates 11/11/2004

There are exercises you can do in your local gym for the legs as long as you are careful not to load up too much weight. In our office, we ask people to work each leg individually to help diagnose if there is a mechanical problem when lifting. If one side is stronger than the other side, it is an indication of mechanical problems that needs addressing by a health care professional. These problems cannot be "exercised" away. By pushing, you will tighten and weaken the problem side.

Quadricep, Hamstring and Abdominal Strengthening Exercises

Quadricep Strengthening. ☐

Prior to performing any exercises on our universal gym, be sure to check and see that the pin is in the desired amount of weight(a). The weight stack for this part of the machine is located to the right of the seat. To strengthen the quadriceps (in front of the thighs), one leg at a time, lift the weight and straighten leg as shown. Begin with 6 repetitions on each side and every other day add 1-2 repetitions (reps) until you reach 18. At that time, increase the weight and begin again with 6 reps and build back up to 18, and then increase the weight again.

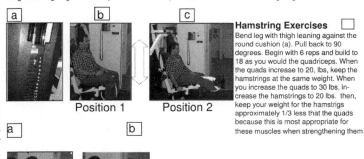

Position 1   Position 2

(c) Copyright, Charschan Chiropractic and Sports Injury Associates 2003

Hamstring Exercises ☐

Bend leg with thigh leaning against the round cushion (a). Pull back to 90 degrees. Begin with 6 reps and build to 18 as you would the quadriceps. When the quads increase to 20, lbs, keep the hamstrings at the same weight. When you increase the quads to 30 lbs, increase the hamstrings to 20 lbs. then, keep your weight for the hamstrigs approximately 1/3 less that the quads because this is most appropriate for these muscles when strengthening them.

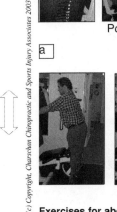
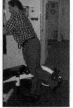

General Rules- If the exercise causes pain, discontinue and tell the doctor. If there is considerable weakness on one side or you cannot do the exercise, let the doctor know. He will help you.

Position 3

Exercises for abdominal muscles ☐

This is a challenging sit-up that can significantly add tone to the region while helping to shape the core muscles. First suck your stomach in (a), flattening your back to the table or floor. Continue contracting these muscles this

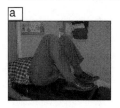
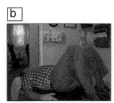

way until the legs begin to lift slightly off the table (b). The goal is to lift the legs using the abdominal muscles only. Begin with 5 reps and increase daily to one set of 15. Then every other day, add a second and then a third set.

To begin adequately strengthening the shoulder girdle you must improve shoulder posture, strengthen the posterior elements in the shoulder joints and then strengthen the actual joints. You should be able to perform these postural and individual shoulder muscle strengthening exercises successfully at home before going to the local gym and using the universal gym equipment. (Available to download at www.backfixer1.com/bookexercises.)

Upper Back Postural Exercises

These exercises are designed to strengthen the posterior upper back mucles that are often neglected. The benefits are a reduction in perceived stress in the shoulders and neck, an improvement in shoulder function and improved breathing. If you are at work and sit behind a desk, perform these periodically throughout the week.

Rhomboid, Middle Trap Exercise. ☐

This exercise will strengthen the rhomboids and mid and upper traps as well. Begin with arms held at 90 degrees, Your goal is to aim your right elbow toward the left pocket and left toward the right. When doing this, your shoulder blades should come together at the black line in illustration. Imagine someone putting a pencil in between your blades and expecting you to hold it there. That is the correct way to perform this. Begin with 3 sets of 10 seconds holding this position, adding an additional set daily until you do 10 sets. Then, every other day, increase the time from 10 seconds to 30, 3 times per week.

Back View   Front View

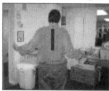   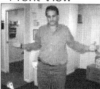

Lower Traps Exercises ☐

Pull the fingertips down toward the floor. Then, with the hands pulling downward (a), rotate the wrists outward (b). Begin with 6 repetitions, and then, every day, increase the repetitions to 18 repetitions. Once you have done this, every other day, increase the repetitions more until you reach 3 sets of 18, three times per week. These muscles, when toned, will also help keep the shoulders back and improve upper back function and improve shoulder strength.

☐

General Stretch and Tone Exercise For Upper Back and Chest.

These exercises are designed to bring the shoulders back and improve posture. In position A, bring hands back as shown until the hands begin to tingle and hold 30 seconds. In position B, bring arms back as shown until fingers begin to tingle and hold 30 seconds. In position C, bring arms back with arms bent at 90 degrees and rotate hands backward until the hands tingle and hold for 30 seconds. These exercises will stretch open the anterior chest muscles and tone the posterior shoulder muscles. Perform periodically during the day to relieve tension and stress and reinforce good posture.

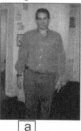

Position A   Position B   Position C

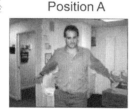   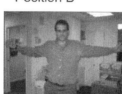

General Rules

If the exercise causes pain, discontinue and tell the doctor. If there is considerable weakness on one side or you cannot do the exercise, let the doctor know. He will help you.

Individual Shoulder Muscle Exercises with Free Weights

All exercises are to be done in one set. Begin with a hand weight of _____lbs. Begin with 10 repetitions and work toward 50 - 60 in one set. Once you have completed your goal, you may either increase the weight or begin working muscle groups..

☐ Anterior Deltoid   ☐ Posterior Deltoid

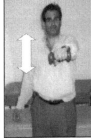 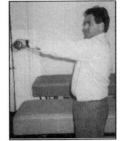 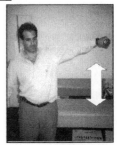

The Deltoids should be exercised by starting in the 90 degree position, going up about 10 - 15 degrees and by going down by the same amount. These are the active ranges of motion of these muscles

Infraspinatis ☐   ☐ Subscapularis

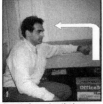 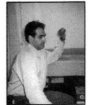 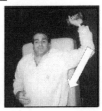

The subscapularis is exercised by resting your shoulder so it sits off the bed. The arm is held at 90 degrees as shown. The exercise is performed by rotation of the arm forward 90 degrees at the fore-arm until it reaches the second position as shown.

The infraspinatis is exercised by resting your elbow on a table and lifting the arm holding the weight to 90 degrees as shown

☐ Teres Minor

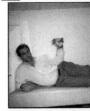 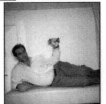 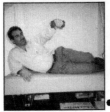 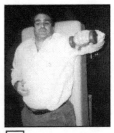

The Teres Minor is exercised by resting your elbow on your side. Lift the weight straight up into the air with the elbow held to your side as shown.

Supraspinatis ☐

The supraspinatis is exercised by laying on your side, placing the arm as shown with your wrist against the table and lifting your arm straight up until it is about 30 degrees above your shoulder as shown.

Dr. William Charschan, Director
490 Georges Rd. North Brunswick
1281 Raritan Rd. Scotch Plains
Charschan Chiropractic
AND SPORTS INJURY ASSOCIATES
(732) 846 - 6400
www.backfixer1.com

Exercises for the Hand and Forearm

Strength is coordinated mechanical advantage. The overall goal of exercises throughout the kinetic chains is to improve the timing and coordination of the muscles so that when you perform 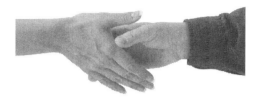 even the simplest tasks, you have much greater strength because of well-coordinated movement. The incorrect alternative is hoping that exercises at the gym will make you stronger. This is why people with many chronic problems continue to exercise and hurt themselves. If the movement were more coordinated, there would be far greater strength gains without injury. It is not how strong an area or part is but rather, how the parts work together as a group to accomplish the task.

When the hand and forearm have loosened up, exercise is necessary to strengthen the tissues and improve movement coordination. Flexible muscles work more efficiently and need exercise to improve their overall function and to establish more favorable movement patterns and free myofascial restrictions. As a rule, when a health care provider loosens adhesions and restores function, even though these regions are working

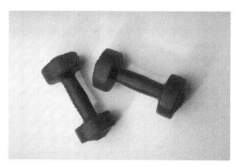 more efficiently, they need to be strengthened for endurance, and better movement needs to be learned to decrease the likelihood that the problem will return over time.

Exercises to the shoulder, forearm and upper arm using one to three pound free weights, available at most sporting goods stores, are very effective in helping to strengthen the region.

Strengthening the biceps and triceps is necessary for increased shoulder efficiency because these muscles affect movement of both the shoulder joint and the elbow. When the biceps and triceps are tight, they prevent proper movement at the elbow and the wrist may strain and hurt. Biceps and triceps exercises with either free weights or a universal gym are effective to improve the tone and strength of these muscles, allowing the forearm to work more effectively during normal tasks such as opening doors and grabbing things.

A few devices are helpful to exercise the forearm. One of the most simple is therapuddy, which comes in different weights, allowing you to squeeze it as you watch television or perform other activities where you are not otherwise using your hands. It is similar to silly putty. You can also use bands designed to put on your fingers that allow you to extend your fingers against the force, strengthening the posterior forearm muscles.

References and Sources

1. http://en.wikipedia.org/wiki/History_of_health_care_reform_in_the_United_States

2. NY Times, February 13th, 2008

3. Powers, Madison. Managed Care: How Economic Incentive Reforms Went Wrong Kennedy Institute of Ethics Journal - Volume 7, Number 4, December 1997, pp. 353-360

4. Medical bills underlie 60 percent of U.S. bankrupts: study Thu Jun 4, 2009 Reuters News Service

5. HR.BLR.com December 23, 2008 Many Employers Report 2009 Health care-Cost Increases of More than 10%

6. http://www.entrepreneur.com/tradejournals/article/200338813.html. Ailing economy has companies cutting back on benefits: health care coverage in greatest jeopardy of reforms, rising costs.

7. http://www.nj.com/news/index.ssf/2008/04/study_nj_hospital_patients_get.html

8. http://blog.nj.com/ledgerarchives/2007/12/high_cost_of_dying.html

9. http://www.nj.com/news/ledger/topstories/index.ssf/2008/06/_hospice6.html

10. http://www.truth-out.org/article/the-new-york-times-the-high-cost-health-care

11. http://www.chiroweb.com/mpacms/dc/article.php?id=36399 . Chiropractors as Primary Care through AMI.

12. http://www.canadianbusiness.com/managing/strategy/article.jsp?content=20101025_10022_10022.

13. http://en.wikipedia.org/wiki/Statins

14. http://www.metamath.com/math124/statis/Marhelio.htm

15. http://www.rxlist.com/tagamet-drug.htm

16. http://www.cancerisafungus.com/

17. http://www.army.mil/usapa/epubs/pdf/r40_501.pdf

18. http://pressroom.consumerreports.org/pressroom/2009/04/consumer-reports-survey-hands-on-therapies-among-top-rated-treatments-for-back-pain.html

19. http://chirobase.org/07Strategy/AHCPR/ahcprclinician.html

20. http://content.healthaffairs.org/cgi/content/full/hlthaff.w3.283v1/DC1

21. http://www.chiroweb.com/mpacms/dc_ca/article.php?id=38675

22. http://www.dynamicchiropractic.com/mpacms/dc/article.php?id=51219

23. The Effectiveness and Cost Effectiveness of Chiropractic Management of Low-Back Pain (The Manga Report). Pran Manga and Associates (1993) - University of Ottawa, Canada.

24. Acute Low Back Problems in Adults. Clinical Practice Guidelines. Bigos S, et al. Agency for Health Care Policy and Research Publication No. 950642 (1994) - U.S. Department of Health and Human Services.

25. Eisenberg, David M., et al. Trends in alternative medicine use in the United States, 1990-1997. Journal of the American Medical Association, Vol. 280, November 11, 1998, pp. 1569-75

26. Diagnosis and Treatment of Low Back Pain: A Joint Clinical Practice Guideline from the American College of Physicians and the American Pain Society. Roger Chou, MD; Amir Qaseem, MD, PhD, MHA; Vincenza Snow, MD; Donald Casey, MD, MPH, MBA; J. Thomas Cross Jr., MD, MPH; Paul Shekelle, MD, PhD; and Douglas K. Owens, MD, MS, for the Clinical Efficacy Assessment Subcommittee of the American College of Physicians and the American College of Physicians/American Pain Society Low Back Pain Guidelines Panel. October 2, 2007vol. 147 no. 7 478-491.

27. http://en.wikipedia.org/wiki/Restless_legs_syndrome

28. http://en.wikipedia.org/wiki/Carotid_endarterectomy

29. http://health.ezinemark.com/brushing-your-teeth-keeps-your-heart-healthy-16bde67cac4.html

30. Screening using whole-body magnetic resonance imaging scanning: who wants an incidentaloma? Rustam Al-Shahi Salman,William NWhiteley, CharlesWarlow J Med Screen 2007;14:2–4.

31. http://www.annals.org/content/149/3/185.full

32. http://www.news.harvard.edu/gazette/2003/09.18/15-foodpyramid.html

33. http://www.who.int/dietphysicalactivity/publications/facts/obesity/en/

34. The Effects of Low-Carbohydrate versus Conventional Weight Loss Diets in Severely Obese Adults: One-Year Follow-up of a Randomized Trial Linda Stern, MD; Nayyar Iqbal, MD; Kathryn L. Chicano, CRNP; Denise A. Daily, RD; Joyce McGrory, CRNP;Monica Williams, BS; Edward J. Gracely, PhD; and Frederick F. Samaha, MD. May 18, 2004vol. 140 no. 10 778-785

35. armypubs.army.mil/epubs/pdf/r40_501.pdf

36. http://www.eswtusa.com/

37. *Arthritis Research & Therapy* 2009, 11:R54 (doi:10.1186/ar2673). This article is online at: http://arthritis-research.com/content/11/2/R54 © 2009 Sicras *et al.*; licensee BioMed Central Ltd.

38. *BMJ* 2002; 325 : 185 doi: 10.1136/bmj.325.7357.185 (Published 27 July 2002).

39. Clinical Bulletin of Myofascial Therapy Vol 2, Number 4 1997 Pgs 71-88.

40. Treatment of Fibromyalgia Syndrome With AntidepressantsA Meta-analysis Winfried Häuser, MD; Kathrin Bernardy, PhD; Nurcan Üçeyler, MD; Claudia Sommer, MD *JAMA.* 2009;301(2):198-209.

41. Alternative medicine; physician-patient relations; primary health care. (J Fam Pract 2000; 49:1121-1130)

42. Lumbar Discography: A Comprehensive Review of Outcome Studies, Diagnostic Accuracy, and Principles Steven P. Cohen, M.D., Thomas M. Larkin, M.D., Steven A. Barna, M.D., William E. Palmer, M.D.,

Andrew C. Hecht, M.D., and Milan P. Stojanovic, M.D. Regional Anesthesia and Pain Medicine Vol. 30 No. 2 March–April 2005

43. **Somatic** Dysfunction in **Osteopathic** Family Medicine - Google Books Result by American College of Osteopathic Family ... - 2006 - Medical – Pgs 94-96 Dartmouth Atlas of health Care 2008 Pgs 20-36.

44. Freedman KB, Bernstein J. The adequacy of medical school education in musculoskeletal medicine. **J Bone and Joint Surg,** 80A:1421-1427. Oct. 1998.

45. Healthnews.com Are Modern Diagnostic Tools Being Overused By: Neomi Heroux Published: Tuesday, 11 November 2008

46. November 14, 2008. NY Times. Why Does U.S. Health Care Cost So Much? (Part I) By Uwe E. Reinhardt

47. How Primary Care Heals Health Disparities.The U.S. health care system needs to focus more general. care and care coordination By Christine Gorman September 28, 2010 26 Scientific American

48. Beattie PF, Myers SP, Stratford P, et al. Associations between patient report of symptoms and anatomic impairment visible on lumbar magnetic resonance imaging. Spine, April 1, 2000:25(7), pp819-28.

49. "Failed back surgery syndrome" Education and debate BMJ 2003; 327 : 985 doi: 10.1136/bmj.327.7421.985 (Published 23 October 2003)

50. http://www.consumerreports.org/health/medical-conditions-treatments/back-pain/overview/back-pain.htm

51. http://www.associatedcontent.com/article/1794404/ibuprofen_warnings_you_should_know.html

52. Tilburt JC, et al "Prescribing 'placebo treatments:' Results of national survey of U.S. internists and rheumatologists" **BMJ** 2008; DOI: 10.1136/bmj.a193821. A Controlled Trial of Arthroscopic Surgery for Osteoarthritis of the Knee J. Bruce Moseley, M.D., Kimberly O'Malley, Ph.D., Nancy J. Petersen, Ph.D., Terri J. Menke, Ph.D., Baruch A. Brody, Ph.D., David H. Kuykendall, Ph.D., John C. Hollingsworth, Dr.P.H., Carol M. Ashton, M.D., M.P.H., and Nelda P. Wray, M.D., M.P.H. Volume 347:81-88, July 11, 2002, Number 2

53. November 14, 2008. NY Times. Why Does U.S. Health Care Cost So Much? (Part I) By Uwe E. Reinhardt

54. Health Care Costs: An Aging Population is Not the Problem Apr 10, 2008 Internet site Economistview.com http://economistsview.typepad.com/economistsview/2008/04/health-care-cos.html

55. Dynamic Chiropractic, Aug 16, 2003 AMA resolves to ensure musculoskeletal training for med students.

56. Effects of Pelvis Asymmetry and Low Back Pain on Trunk Kinematics During Sitting: A Comparison With Standing. Einas A Eisa PHD, David Egan PHD, Kevin Deluzio PHD and Richard Wassersug PHD. Spine Vol 31 #5 PP E135-E143.

57. Beattie PF, Myers SP, Stratford P, et al. Associations between patient report of symptoms and anatomic impairment visible on lumbar magnetic resonance imaging. Spine, April 1, 2000:25(7), pp819-28.

58. Neurosurg Clin N Am. 1991 Oct;2(4):899-919. Failed back surgery syndrome. Long DM.Department of Neurological Surgery, Johns Hopkins Hospital, Baltimore, Maryland.

59. http://www.nytimes.com/2008/02/13/health/research/13spine.html

60. Spine J. 2005 Mar-Apr;5(2):191-201.Epidural steroid therapy for back and leg pain: mechanisms of action and efficacy.McLain RF, Kapural L, Mekhail NA. The Cleveland Clinic Spine Institute, The Cleveland Clinic Foundation, 9500 Euclid Avenue, Cleveland, OH 44195, USA. mclainr@ccf.org.

61. Orthopedic Physical Assessment [Hardcover]David J. Magee PhD BPT Saunders; 5 edition (December 10, 2007)

62. The correlation between pes planus and anterior knee or intermittent low back pain.Kosashvili Y, Fridman T, Backstein D, Safir O, Bar Ziv Foot Ankle Int. 2008 Sep;29(9):910-3.Y.Division of Orthopedics, Assaf Harofeh Medical Center, Israel. yonasofi@gmail.com

63. *Knee Injury Patterns Among Men and Women in Collegiate Basketball and Soccer* Elizabeth Arendt, MD, and Randall Dick, MS American Journal of Sports Medicine, Vol. 23, No. 6, 1995

64. Am Fam Physician. 2010 Oct 15;82(8):917-22. Anterior cruciate ligament injury: diagnosis, management, and prevention.Cimino F, Volk BS, *Setter D.*

65. Acta Obstet Gynecol Scand. 2010 Sep;89(9):1187-91.Clinical findings, pain descriptions and physical complaints reported by women with post-natal pregnancy-related pelvic girdle pain. Nielsen LL.Department of Public Health and Primary Health Care, University of Bergen, Norway. Lars.Lennart.Nielsen@fys.no.

66. Mil Med. 2010 May;175(5):329-35. Selected static anatomic measures predict overuse injuries in female recruits. Rauh MJ, Macera CA, Trone DW, Reis JP, Shaffer RA. Naval Health Research Center, 140 Sylvester Road, San Diego, CA 92106-3521, USA.

67. Coccygectomy: an effective treatment option for chronic coccydynia: retrospective results in 41 consecutive patients. Trollegaard AM, Aarby NS, Hellberg S.J Bone Joint Surg Br. 2010 Feb;92(2):242-5. PMID: 20130316

68. Conservative management of sports injuries pages 501-502 by Thomas E. Hyde D.C.D.A.C.B.S.P., Marianne S. Gengenbach D.C.D.A.C.B.S.P (C) 1997 Williams and Wilkins.

69. Weishaupt D et al. "MRI of the lumbar spine: Prevalence of intervertebral disc extrusion and sequestration, nerve root compression and plate abnormalities, and osteoarthritis of the fact joints in Asymptomatic Volunteers." Radiology – 1998; 209:661-666

70. Jensen MC, et al. "MRI imaging of the lumbar spine in people without back pain." N Engl J Med – 1994; 331:369-373

71. Powell MC, et al. "Prevalence of lumbar disc degeneration observed by magnetic resonance in symptomless women." Lancer – 1986; 2:1366-7

72. Coppes NH, et al. "Innervation of anulus fibrosus in Low Back Pain." Lancet 1990; 336:189-190

73. Yochum and Rowe's Essentials of Skeletal Radiology Pg 530-531. (c) 2005 Lippincott Williams and Wilkins.

74. Musculofascial lengthening for the treatment of patients with medial epicondylitis and coexistent ulnar neuropathy.Gong HS, Chung MS,

Kang ES, Oh JH, Lee YH, Baek GH.J Bone Joint Surg Br. 2010 Jun;92(6):823-7.

75. Comparative study of surgical treatment of ulnar nerve compression at the elbow. Mitsionis GI, Manoudis GN, Paschos NK, Korompilias AV, Beris AE.J Shoulder Elbow Surg. 2010 Jun;19(4):513-9. Epub 2010 Feb 10.

76. BMC Musculoskelet Disord. 2010 Nov 30;11(1):275. Bias in the Physical Examination of Patients with Lumbar Radiculopathy.Suri P, Hunter DJ, Katz JN, Li L, Rainville J.

77. Results of an integral lifestyle modification program to reduce weight among overweight and obese women.]Fuentes L L, Muñoz AA.Rev Med Chil. 2010 Aug;138(8):974-981. Epub 2010 Nov 26. Spanish.

78. http://www.who.int/dietphysicalactivity/publications/facts/obesity/en/index.html.

79. Effects of glucosamine, chondroitin, or placebo in patients with osteoarthritis of hip or knee: network meta-analysis. Wandel S, Jüni P, Tendal B, Nüesch E, Villiger PM, Welton NJ, Reichenbach S, Trelle S. BMJ. 2010 Sep 16;341:c4675. doi: 10.1136/bmj.c4675.

80. www.ncbi.nlm.nih.gov/pmc/articles/.../pdf/canmedaj01499-0102.pdf

81. Chiropractic manipulation in Adolescent Idiopathic Scoliosis: a pilot study **Dale E Rowe, Ronald J Feise2, Edward R Crowther, Jaroslaw P Grod, J Michael Menke, Charles H Goldsmith, Michael R Stoline, Thomas A Souzaand Brandon Kambach** *Chiropractic & Osteopathy* 2006, 14:15 doi:10.1186/1746-1340-14-15

82. http://runningtimes.com/Article.aspx?ArticleID=3858&PageNum=2

83. Chakravarty EF, Hubert HB, Lingala VB, Zatarain E, Fries JF. Long distance running and knee osteoarthritis. A prospective study. American Journal of Preventive Medicine 2008 Aug;35(2):133-8

About the Author

Since 1988, Dr. William D. Charschan, D.C., CCSP has treated more than thousands of patients in New Jersey suffering from accident trauma, occupational stress injuries, sports injuries and chronic pain associated with the simplest everyday activities and aging.

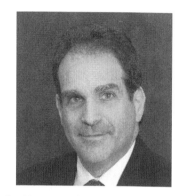

A graduate of the National College of Chiropractic (now known as the National College of Health Sciences) located in Lombard, Illinois; Dr. Charschan also received his certification in sports injuries in 1991 at New York Chiropractic College. A Certified Sports Physician and the Medical Director for USA Track and Field New Jersey, Dr. Charschan is a licensed and board certified physician of chiropractic medicine with a background in mechanical engineering.

Dr. Charschan is an avid explorer of safe, non-surgical, results-oriented patient care and studied soft tissue and myofascial release treatments taught by maverick men of chiropractic medicine, Doctors Warren Hammer (**Fascial Manipulation**© www. fascialmanipulationworkshops.com) and Michael Leahy (Active Release Techniques®). He studied the Graston Technique method of soft tissue treatment and its application in addressing chronic pain syndromes and is trained in orthotics theory and application by Len Kerns of Foot Function lab.

Focusing on the biomechanics of running and gait, Dr. Charschan is passionate about the need for a system that allows health care practitioners to better diagnose, agree and then treat mechanical problems, the basis for most chronic pain. Building on the work of Dr. Brian Rothbart, Dr. Charschan developed unique methods of screening body mechanics based on body style in a way that makes it easy to improve diagnostic inter reliability between health care practitioners.

Dr. Charschan has lectured on his diagnostic methods and treatment to the sports council at Palmer Chiropractic College, Association of NJ Chiropractors Sports Council and has published articles on kinetic chains in the magazine *Dynamic Chiropractic*.

Dr. Charschan regularly volunteers at numerous athletic events including track and field, Marshal Arts, Ultimate Frisbee, National Aerobic championships, Grappling, Soccer, Football and The New York marathon.

Practicing in Scotch Plains and North Brunswick, Dr. Charschan lives in New Jersey with his wonderful wife Beth, a business owner, his daughter, Gabriell, and son, Jesse who is glad to have a chiropractor for a dad after an afternoon of raking fall leaves.

Visit www.backfixer1.com for information.